best of
Choice Menus

MEAL PLANNING AND RECIPES FOR DIABETES AND HEALTHY EATING

MARJORIE ANDERSON HOLLANDS AND MARGARET HOWARD

Know who to turn to

 CANADIAN DIABETES ASSOCIATION | ASSOCIATION CANADIENNE DU DIABÈTE

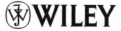 **WILEY**

John Wiley & Sons Canada, Ltd.

National Library of Canada Cataloguing in Publication

Hollands, Marjorie, 1930-
    Best of choice menus [text (large print)] : diabetic cooking and meal planning for the visually challenged / Marjorie Hollands, Margaret Howard.

Includes index.
ISBN 0-470-83442-0

    1. Diabetes--Diet therapy--Recipes. 2. Large type books.
I. Howard, Margaret, 1930- II. Title.

RC662.H638 2004   641.5'6314   C2003-907385-8

Production Credits
Cover & interior text design: Interrobang Graphic Design Inc.
Cover photo credit: Getty Images / Bruce James / Vine Ripe Tomatoes
Printer: Tri-Graphic Printing Ltd.
Printed in Canada
10 9 8 7 6 5 4 3 2 1

contents

acknowledgements

To all those readers with vision impairment, we thank you. You were the inspiration for this larger print edition of the *Choice Menus* series.

To those who supplied counsel and guidance in the preparation of this book: Sharon Zeiler of The Canadian Diabetes Association (CDA) and Linda Studholme of the Canadian National Institute for the Blind (CNIB).

A special thank you to the dedicated dietitians and diabetes educators who reviewed the manuscript ensuring its accuracy: Linda Aurnell, Nicole Aylward, Deidre Barker, Beverley Harris, Rebecca Horsman and Michelle Knezic.

To Sharyn Joliat of Info Access (1988) Inc. for her expert nutritional analysis and verification of food choice values for the revised recipes used in this book.

A special thanks to Dr. Anne Kenshole, former Medical Director of TRIDEC (Tri-Hospital Diabetes Education Centre) at Sunnybrook and Women's College Health Science Centre, Toronto, for writing the foreword to this book.

To our many friends at John Wiley & Sons Canada, Ltd., for their cooperation and support.

 To the many graduates of TRIDEC, your requests for "a month of menus" were the reason we wrote the original *Choice Menus* series.

To Marian Hebb and Monique van Remortel, for their legal counsel, to John Howard for expert editorial advice and to our families for their ongoing support and encouragement.

foreword

What this is *not* is yet another "diet book." Instead, you will find within its pages plenty of good ideas about meal planning, together with recipes that are based on sound nutritional principles and which can be enjoyed by the whole family or served to guests with pride.

Eating balanced meals plays a vital role in the successful management of diabetes. Moreover, good eating is just as important in weight control and the prevention of diabetes.

This larger print edition has been specifically designed to help people with impaired vision to continue to enjoy one of life's greatest and enduring pleasures—the pleasure of the table!

Dr. Anne Kenshole,
Past Medical Director, Tri-Hospital Diabetes Education Centre
Sunnybrook and Women's College Health Science Centre
Emeritus Professor of Medicine, University of Toronto

general introduction

Our goal in the *Choice Menus* cookbook series has always been to simplify meal planning and to promote weight control, especially for those with type 2 diabetes. However, many readers have told us they could read the print in *Choice Menus* easily, but now they don't see as well as they used to and need a larger print. So we have chosen favourite menus and recipes from our previous three books—*Choice Menus, More Choice Menus* and *Choice Menus Presents*—and published them in a larger print version—*Best of Choice Menus*.

We believe our Choice Menus series has an important role to play in the ongoing battle with diabetes, both in management and prevention. Over 2 million Canadians have diabetes (although three out of ten don't know it) with an estimated 60,000 new cases diagnosed every year. Of those diagnosed, 90 percent have type 2 diabetes and 10 percent have type 1.

The Importance of Meal Planning

Maybe you don't have diabetes, but you'd like to lose some weight. Maybe you've been thinking it's time to improve your eating habits and are looking for some direction. Whatever your goal, planning healthy meals is of utmost importance. A healthier lifestyle helps you feel better and have more energy and it decreases your risk for chronic diseases such as diabetes, cancer and heart disease.

When it comes to the person with diabetes, diet is still the cornerstone of good management. Careful meal planning has never been more important. Research makes it clear that keeping blood glucose levels close to normal can prevent and possibly delay the complications of diabetes. The person with type 1 diabetes needs to balance carbohydrate intake with insulin and exercise to achieve good control. For those with type 2 diabetes, attention to food portions and physical activity is the most direct route to a healthy weight and better diabetes control. In both cases we're talking *what* to eat, *how much* to eat and even *when* to eat.

If you are overweight and have type 2 diabetes, changing lifestyle will promote a healthier body weight. Even a weight loss of 10 lbs (4.5 kg) can result in better diabetes control. Combining healthy eating with daily exercise like walking will help achieve even better diabetes control.

If you are a lean person with type 2 diabetes, you do not want to lose any more weight, but you do need to carefully balance your food intake with your available insulin supply. Planning five or six small meals over the day is one strategy.

If you have type 1 diabetes, your insulin action may need a slightly different meal pattern than is used in our menus. Ask your dietitian or diabetes educator for advice. However, you will find *Best of Choice Menus* a useful resource to use with your meal plan. The menus can provide inspiration and the Food Choice values given with each recipe make it easy to use them in any meal plan.

Maybe you don't have diabetes—but there is a history of diabetes in your family—and you've been thinking that you really should lose some weight and improve your eating habits. Let our menus be your guide. *Best of Choice Menus* offers a month of healthy and tasty menus for breakfast, lunch and dinner, plus snacks that you can mix and match to your individual eating style. Many menus are simple and quickly prepared. Others take more time and may be ones you'll choose when you are cooking for family or guests. Many need no special recipes. Other menus include wonderful new recipes we know will become family favourites. All the menus are based on the Canadian Diabetes Association food choice system of meal planning and are planned especially for someone with type 2 diabetes. For more, see "How To Use This Book" (page 11).

Our menus do not replace nutritional counselling from a registered dietitian. You are an individual, with your own food preferences and lifestyle. A dietitian can help you identify problem areas and set realistic goals, then work with you to prepare an individualized meal plan. You will also need ongoing support and encouragement and someone to answer questions as they arise, but our menus and recipes are always there to give variety and fresh ideas.

Variety, Moderation and Balance

Canada's Food Guide to Healthy Eating has three key healthy messages: *variety*, *moderation* and *balance*. These nutrition principles apply to people with diabetes as much as they do to other Canadians.

- Enjoy a variety of foods from each food group each day.
- Choose whole-grain and enriched products more often.
- Choose dark green and orange vegetables and orange fruit more often.
- Choose lower-fat milk products more often.
- Choose leaner meats, poultry and fish, as well as dried peas, beans and lentils more often.

When you choose daily menus like these in *Best of Choice Menus*, you know you are getting a variety of healthy foods in moderate portions in balanced meals spaced over the day—and that's eating well. We believe that eating a variety of healthy foods is a more effective and enjoyable way to good health than the routine use of nutritional supplements.

The Canadian Diabetes Association's *Good Health Eating Guide* emphasizes overall food intake. *What*, *how much* and even *how often* are important to good health. Both guides emphasize there are no "good" foods or "bad" foods. All foods can be part of a healthy diet. The secret is moderation and balance.

Guidelines for the Nutritional Management of Diabetes

The National Nutrition Committee of the Canadian Diabetes Association publishes guidelines for diabetes and healthy eating every few years based on current research on food and diabetes. The *Choice Menus* series and *Best of Choice Menus* follow these guidelines.

The current guidelines stress the importance of normal blood glucose and cholesterol levels as well as the importance of healthy eating and a healthy weight. With the increasing use of glucose monitors to measure blood glucose before and after meals, it is now possible to fine-tune meal plans and medication to preferences and lifestyle in a way that was not possible ten or fifteen years ago.

Carbohydrates

The carbohydrate family includes all forms of starch and sugar. Digestion releases starch and sugar from foods and breaks them down into glucose, the simplest form of sugar and our main source of energy. Glucose passes into the bloodstream after meals, resulting in a rise in blood glucose (or blood sugar) and a release of insulin hormone by the pancreas. The total amount of carbohydrate you eat at a meal is very important. At one time it was thought that sugars raised blood glucose quickly and starches raised it more slowly. However, it is clear now that this was far too simple an approach and recent research shows that there are other factors that decide how quickly or slowly blood glucose rises after a meal. Some of these are:

- *Food form*. Drinking a glass of fruit juice will raise the blood glucose more quickly than eating a solid whole fruit.

- *Degree of processing*. The starch in a highly processed breakfast cereal such as cornflakes digests faster than the starch in a whole grain cereal such as oatmeal.

- *Cooking method*. Starch in a mashed potato digests more rapidly than starch in a boiled or baked potato.

Surge Protection

Since insulin tends to be released slowly in type 2 diabetes, it is important to plan meals that will raise blood glucose gradually. Nutrition research has identified several things you can do to help slow the rise or surge in blood glucose after a meal. Menus and recipes in the *Choice Menus* series have been planned with these in mind.

- Eat carbohydrate foods as part of a *mixed meal*, one that contains protein and fat as well as fibre. Animal or vegetable protein and fats or oils digest very slowly and slow the digestion of the starches and sugars eaten with them. However, an excessive amount of fat or oil in a meal can make it difficult for the insulin supply to work effectively. So can too much carbohydrate at one meal. Moderation and balance are the secret.

- Choose carbohydrate-containing foods that *digest slowly*. Fruits and vegetables rich in fibre take longer to digest than do their juices; foods containing soluble sticky fibre (oats, barley, legumes, pectin), as well as insoluble bran fibre, digest even more slowly.

- *Space meals* at regular intervals throughout the day to make better use of a limited insulin supply. Skipping meals, then overeating at the next meal, is not a good idea. Research has shown that spreading food over several small meals a day can result in better blood glucose and cholesterol values after meals (see "Snacks", page 167).

- Limit the *amount of starch and sugar* you eat at each meal. This is most important if you are to achieve improved blood glucose control. You need a certain amount of carbohydrate in each meal to encourage your pancreas to produce insulin. But too much starch or sugar may be too much for your insulin supply to handle. Balance and moderation are again the key.

Glycemic Index

Much new information about food and diabetes comes from *glycemic index* (GI) research. This research compares the effects that different starchy foods have on blood glucose in the same individual. Quickly digested foods, such as white bread, have a high glycemic index; they raise blood glucose rapidly. Unrefined, more slowly digested foods, such as legumes, barley, pasta and oats, have a lower glycemic index; they raise blood glucose more slowly and gradually. The use of low GI foods helps improve diabetes control and also helps reduce the risk of developing type 2 diabetes. Our menus and recipes use lower glycemic index foods wherever possible.

The following table illustrates how different foods with the same carbohydrate content are rated.

Low GI Foods *Choose most often*	Medium GI Foods *Choose more often*	High GI Foods *Choose less often*
BREADS 100% stone ground whole wheat bread heavy multigrain bread pumpernickel bread	BREADS whole wheat bread rye bread pita bread	BREADS white bread kaiser roll bagel, white
CEREAL All Bran™ Bran Buds with Psyllium™ oatmeal oat bran	CEREAL shredded wheat quick oats	CEREAL bran flakes corn flakes Rice Krispies™ Cheerios™
GRAINS parboiled/converted rice barley bulgar couscous pasta/noodles	GRAINS basmati rice brown rice	GRAINS short grain rice
OTHER sweet potatoes/yams lentils chick peas kidney beans split peas soybeans baked beans	OTHER sweet corn popcorn Ryvita™ (rye crisps) Stoned Wheat Thins™ black bean soup green pea soup	OTHER baking potato french fries pretzels rice cakes soda crackers

Source: CDA 2003 Clinical Practice Guidelines for the Prevention and Management of Diabetes in Canada.

Sugars

Previous guidelines limited the use of sugar from all sources. However, current guidelines recommend including naturally occurring sugars from fruits, vegetables and milk products in meals. Table forms of sugar are permissible in limited amounts. The *total amount of carbohydrate* eaten in a meal is considered more important than whether or not a food contains sugar. Our recipes call for a variety of nutritive and non-nutritive sweeteners. Sugar is used in some recipes, but in small amounts, and counts as part of the carbohydrate in that meal.

In our menu sections, each meal contains a consistent planned amount of carbohydrate, less at breakfast and more at lunch and dinner. Snacks vary in carbohydrate content according to size (see page 15 for details).

Fibre

Everyone, including people with diabetes, should eat more dietary fibre. Increasing fibre intake may reduce risk of coronary heart disease by lowering serum cholesterol in the blood and may reduce risk of type 2 diabetes as well. The soluble fibre in oats, fruit, legumes and barley, as well as the insoluble fibre in wheat bran and the outer peel of fruits and vegetables, slow digestion and thus the rise in blood glucose after a meal.

We pay special attention to fibre in our recipes and menus. All recipes list fibre content. We include high-fibre foods in menus whenever possible.

Protein

People with diabetes do not need any more (or less) protein than those without diabetes, but the guidelines do suggest that excessive intake should be avoided. However, anyone following a weight-loss plan must be sure to get enough protein, as must vegetarians. Some evidence suggests that vegetable protein may be better for reducing serum cholesterol and managing proteinuria. Vegetarians must find alternatives to meats. This can be difficult to manage with the carbohydrate restrictions of diabetes and needs expert knowledge and assistance.

Fats and Oils

Many studies indicate that high-fat diets can impair glucose tolerance and promote obesity, high cholesterol levels and heart disease. When saturated fat is reduced, all these problems reverse or improve. Thus, the emphasis continues to be on reducing intake of *saturated fat* in meat, poultry and dairy products by choosing lower fat foods more often. And there is new emphasis in the current guidelines on limiting intake of processed foods containing *trans-fatty acids* (the fat found in hydrogenated vegetable oil shortening and hard margarine used in many commercial snacks and baked products). This fat may be even more harmful than saturated fat since it not only raises "bad" LDL cholesterol values but also lowers "good" HDL cholesterol.

Some fats are better for diabetes than others. *Omega-3 fats*, found in fatty fish (see page 230), are linked to heart health and may reduce serum triglyceride, a type of blood fat often elevated in diabetes. For that reason, the current guidelines recommend eating fish, such as salmon or sardines, at least once or twice a week.

Research indicates that *monounsaturated fats* (such as canola and olive oils) may have a beneficial effect on both triglycerides and glycemic control. Current guidelines recommend that these oils and the soft non-hydrogenated margarine made from them be used in small amounts to avoid weight gain. Our recipes and menus reflect these guidelines.

Sodium and Hypertension

It is important to keep hypertension (or high blood pressure) under control, especially if you have Type 2 diabetes. Attaining a healthier weight through balanced eating and regular physical activity is often enough to normalize blood pressure. Guidelines also advise avoiding or limiting alcohol and smoking to reduce blood pressure. Keeping sodium intake down (2000–4000 mg per day) may also benefit those with hypertension. Our recipes give the sodium content per serving as well as many tips on how to reduce salt intake.

Carbohydrate Counting

Research evidence suggests that persons with a consistent carbohydrate intake (that eat about the same amount of carbohydrate at each meal) find it easier to keep blood glucose near normal. Many people with diabetes use carbohydrate counting in meal planning. They set carbohydrate goals for each meal, then learn how to count the amount they eat at each meal. They do this either by memorizing food values or by using the *Good Health Eating Guide* (see below). However, since the focus is on carbohydrate, they must also take care to eat healthy meals.

Each of our menus is based on a planned amount of carbohydrate (see Appendix 6, page 238) and is nutritionally balanced. We have included weights and measures in both menus and recipes wherever we thought they would be useful, especially for high-carbohydrate foods. This should help the "carb counters" keep their carbohydrate intake planned and consistent.

The Good Health Eating Guide (GHEG)

Another approach to meal planning used by many people with diabetes is the GHEG developed by the Canadian Diabetes Association. It is a system based on Canada's Food Guide to Healthy Eating (see page 226) adapted to the needs of a diabetes meal plan. Foods are divided into different groups according to the amount of carbohydrate, protein and fat they contain. A serving of a food is described as a CHOICE, since it *is* your choice. By choosing a variety of foods from each group at each meal, you're sure to get all the nutrients you need, as well as having balanced meals and a consistent carbohydrate intake.

Each of our recipes includes Food Choice values as well as a nutritional analysis. Each of our menus is planned to fit into the food choices of the meal plan shown on page 15. For more about the GHEG, see Appendix 2, page 226.

What's Next?

Future research will no doubt discover new information about food and diabetes. However, we happen to believe that healthy meals that include a wide variety of vegetables, fruits, grains and high-fibre starchy foods, along with low-fat protein foods and milk products, will continue to get top priority.

Meal Planning Tips

We have worked hard to streamline each recipe so you can minimize time spent in the kitchen but still make meals from scratch. The recipes in this book are basically simple. Most take no longer than 30 minutes to prepare. We have tried to use ingredients that are readily available. Naturally those of you who are familiar with the format of our other books will remember that menus are the basis of these books, so we emphasize that *each menu describes one serving*. Sometimes you will be cooking for several people, and other times for just one or two. To help you in your choice of menu, each recipe used in a menu shows how many it serves (1/2 serves two people; 1/6 serves six people).

Low-Vision Meal Planning Tips

Healthy eating is important for everyone. Your meal plan, *Best of Choice Menus* and the *Good Health Eating Guide* are your best resources.

Here are some suggestions from friends with low vision as well as from the Canadian National Institute for the Blind (CNIB) to make life a little bit easier.

Shopping Tips

The key to efficient food shopping is thinking ahead and doing effective meal planning. Shopping should be as infrequent and as complete as possible other than for fresh produce. To do this, plan ahead to know what you need to buy. With *Best of Choice Menus*, you have all the answers. The meal planning process then goes like this:

- Start by choosing the menus you intend to use. A week of menus is a good way to begin.

- Make a list of the groceries you must buy for the chosen menus.

- Use a black marker on white for your grocery list to make it easier to read. Organize the list by store sections (for example, dairy, meat, produce, etc.) whether you are shopping in person, by telephone or on-line.

- A small magnifying glass and a penlight will help when reading labels and prices in the store.

Equipment Tips

- A toaster oven and microwave are very useful. Special pads can be applied to microwave controls to allow cooking by touch. Remember to use only microwave-safe dishes when cooking in your microwave oven.

- Small saucepans and ovenproof dishes are good to have on hand. Freezer-to-oven-to-table dishes are also extremely useful.

- Dark cooking pans against a white stove provides contrast. Place pans on the centre of the element with handles turned toward the centre of the stove for safety.

- A few marbles in the bottom of a double boiler will rattle if the water boils away.

- Mark stovetop and oven controls with small strips of contrasting tape. Location dots and hi-marks are available at CNIB.

- Develop the habit of turning the burner or oven off before removing pans.

- Long, flame-resistant oven mitts can prevent accidental burns.

Cooking Tips

- Good lighting helps a great deal, especially in the kitchen. So does colour contrast.

- Mixing bowls in a colour that contrasts with the countertop are more visible.

- A damp dishcloth placed under bowls and pans prevents slipping.

- Read your chosen menu and recipes carefully. Note cooking times, as these are important factors in determining when to do things.

- Simple homemade labels help you identify spice jars and food tins in the cupboard.

- Use a tray to organize ingredients and other items. A raised edge makes the tray easy to clean up afterwards.

- An ice cream scoop can help when measuring batter for pancakes or into muffin tins.

- Chop ingredients and have them all ready before turning on the stove.

- When meat needs browning, do this while vegetables are cooking. Then all will be ready at the same time.

- Prepare a salad and set the table while the main meal is cooking. Salads can be tossed easily in a clean plastic bag. Then simply discard the bag.

- Clean up as you go to reduce cleanup time at the end of the meal. Put away used items.

- Do batch cooking—make your favourite soup, stew, casserole or baked item, then freeze in serving-size portions. Label and date all items with a permanent marker. The freezer manages to make things look totally unfamiliar.

At-the-Table Tips

- Keep a magnifying glass, a small diet scale and *Best of Choice Menus* (open at the menu you have chosen) handy on your kitchen counter at mealtime.

- Use easy-to-identify graduated measures (see page 97) when serving food on your plate.

- Light-coloured plates will show up better against a dark placemat or tabletop. Dark plates show up better against a light background. Similarly, light-coloured food will show up better on a black dish, dark food on a light dish.

- If you set your place at the table the same way every day, you know what to expect. Drinking glass on the right, salt and pepper on the left.

- You can do the same thing with the food on your plate. Use the clock method to place food on your plate: potatoes at 1 o'clock, meat at 6 o'clock to make cutting easier, vegetables at 9 o'clock. A little planning can make mealtime more enjoyable and spill-free.

how to use this book

In the sections that follow, you will find thirty healthy breakfast menus, thirty appetizing lunches, thirty delectable dinner menus and a variety of snacks in different shapes and sizes to fill the gap between meals. Any breakfast menu you choose, plus any lunch menu, plus your choice of dinner menu will add up to about 1200 calories. Then add in one or more snacks during the day to fit your lifestyle and energy needs (see page 15 for carbohydrate and calorie content of meals and snacks).

First, decide *how many calories* you want your meals to provide each day. Are you trying to trim away a few extra pounds? Or do you simply want to maintain your present healthy weight? Your age, sex, body metabolism and active or inactive lifestyle determine how many calories of food energy you use each day. No two people are alike, so it is difficult to say exactly how much you need. Ask your dietitian if you're not sure.

The table below (based on Canada's Nutrition Recommendations, 1990) shows average energy needs at different stages in life.

AVERAGE ENERGY REQUIREMENTS
(calories needed per day)

Age	Sex	To Maintain Weight	To Lose Weight
25–49	M	2700	2200–2400
	F	1900	1400–1600
50–74	M	2300	1800–2000
	F	1800	1300–1500
75 and over	M	2000	1500–1700
	F	1700	1200–1500

The **snack** menus in the "Snack" section (page 169) come in three different sizes:
    75 calories when you just want a bite
    150 calories to fit in mid-morning or afternoon or as a bedtime snack
    300 calorie ones that are really small meals, great for snacks on active days

For **1200** calories: Choose three meals (any breakfast, lunch and dinner)

For **1500** calories: Choose three meals plus two 150-calorie snacks
    OR three meals and one 300-calorie snack
    OR three meals and two 75-calorie snacks and one 150-calorie snack

For **1800** calories: Choose three meals plus two 300-calorie snacks
    OR three meals, two 150-calorie snacks and one 300-calorie snack

For **2100** calories: Choose three meals plus three 300-calorie snacks
    OR any combination that appeals to you

When you eat is up to you and what's convenient. Most people find that spacing meals at intervals over the day helps keep energy levels high and hunger pangs low. This pattern of eating also helps you avoid hypoglycemia or low blood sugar, which is often a concern if you are on medication for diabetes.

When meals are more than four or five hours apart, snacks come in handy. A planned snack is better than an unplanned snack! Ask a dietitian to help you map out a meal plan based on your usual day's routine. If weekends are a lot different than weekdays, you may want to have another plan in mind for weekends. If you work different shifts, many people find it makes life simpler to have a plan in mind for each shift worked, as well as one for days off.

Everyone's different! Blood glucose monitoring may suggest that the amount of carbohydrate in the breakfast menus is a little too much for you and your insulin supply. No problem—just save part of breakfast, eat it a couple of hours later and call it a snack.

a month of menus

This book has a section for each meal—breakfast, lunch, dinner, snacks and special occasions. At the beginning of each section, you will find a month of menus for that meal. You probably won't use the menus in sequence, although we tried to plan them to avoid repeating the same foods—except when we knew you'd have leftovers on hand. You will, no doubt, find favourite menus to repeat over and over, or you may have the same breakfast two or three days in a row. It's your choice!

Food Is One of Life's Great Pleasures

We believe that mealtimes should be high points in your day. To prove this, *Best of Choice Menus* brings you a month of nutritious—and delicious—meal ideas and over 100 time-tested recipes. As before, some meals are simpler and easier to prepare. Others take longer. Some menus need recipes; others do not. Many dishes can be prepared ahead; others are last-minute. Most of the first menus you come to in a section need no special recipes or only simple ones described in the menus themselves. Other menus call for the more detailed recipes that follow.

Rather than grouping recipes as in a traditional cookbook, we have grouped recipes according to the meals in which they are used. So you'll find a "Breakfast" chapter, a "Lunch" chapter, a "Dinner" chapter and a "Snacks" chapter with information about the importance of that meal and tips for healthy meal planning. That way, all the recipes you need in a menu are there side-by-side for easier use. When you're planning a meal for company, remember the "Special Occasions" chapter (page 195)—with wonderful menus and recipes for entertaining—and each menu still fits into a diabetes meal plan, with the same amount of carbohydrate (although a few more calories!).

We hope this larger print edition makes life a little simpler for you by taking some of the guesswork out of meal planning, by helping you plan varied, delicious and healthy meals that are both good for you and good-tasting. We firmly believe that eating well results in better total health. Enjoy!

Marjorie Hollands and Margaret Howard
March 2004

food choice values of menus

breakfast

- **Each BREAKFAST MENU provides about 330 calories and is based on:**

  2 STARCH CHOICES
  1 FRUITS & VEGETABLES CHOICE
  1 MILK (1%) CHOICE
  1 PROTEIN CHOICE
  1 FATS & OILS CHOICE

lunch

- **Each LUNCH MENU provides about 430 calories and is based on:**

  2 STARCH CHOICES
  2 FRUITS & VEGETABLES CHOICES
  1 MILK (1%) CHOICE
  2 PROTEIN CHOICES
  1 FATS & OILS CHOICE
  1 EXTRA

dinner

- **Each DINNER MENU provides about 500 calories and is based on:**

  2 STARCH CHOICES
  2 FRUITS & VEGETABLES CHOICES
  1 MILK (1%) CHOICE
  3 PROTEIN CHOICES
  1 FATS & OILS CHOICE
  1 EXTRA

snacks

- **SNACK MENUS provide either:**

  75 calories (with 10–15 g carbohydrate)

  OR 150 calories (with 15–20 g carbohydrate)

  OR 300 calories (with 35–40 g carbohydrate)

breakfast

The Importance of Breakfast

Did you know the word "breakfast" comes from *break* (meaning to stop or interrupt) and *fast* (meaning to go without food)? How apt! By morning, having fasted for eight to twelve hours, the average person's brain and muscles need a fresh supply of glucose energy. Eating a balanced breakfast helps your body refuel. Furthermore, studies show that breakfast eaters consume less fat and more nutrients each day than breakfast skippers. A healthy breakfast is truly a healthy start to the day.

Those of you who have diabetes should not even think about skipping breakfast! If you have Type 2 diabetes, you may have noticed your blood glucose is often higher before breakfast than before other meals—and eating breakfast helps bring it back to more normal levels.

Over and above the health aspects of breakfast, this first meal of the day can be an experience rich in flavours and variety. Our recipes and menus will help you achieve a great breakfast cuisine that is both enjoyable and healthy.

Breakfast Strategies

1. Make breakfast so exciting that you could never think of missing it. We believe no one would ever think of missing any of the breakfasts in this section.

2. Plan breakfasts for the time available. Weekends are a perfect time for leisurely breakfasts. Family members can make and eat breakfast at a more relaxed pace. But weekdays are another matter. Time is often short as families go off in all directions.

3. Night-before organization reduces the morning breakfast panic. Any or all of the following can be done the night before:

   - Set the table along with any non-perishable breakfast items.

   - Plan coffee preparation, maybe with an automatic timer.

   - Make a fruit shake and store in the refrigerator (see menu #21).

   - Have ready-to-eat cold cereals handy.

   - Organize hot cereals for the microwave (see menus #14, #18 and #24).

Fruit or Juice?

"Eat your fruit, don't drink it" is a good motto to follow. Fruit juices are a source of vitamins and minerals but valuable fibre has been lost during processing. Raw fruits contain the same vitamins, but also contain insoluble fibre and often soluble fibre as well. Since it takes more time to digest the fibre in raw fruit, the fruit's natural sugar is released more slowly and gradually than when you drink the juice. This, in turn, results in a slower and more gradual increase in your blood glucose levels. And there is an additional dividend. You'll feel more satisfied after eating a piece of fruit than after drinking a glass of juice. If you do have a small glass of juice on occasion, sip it slowly.

Cereals

Cereals are the foundation of a healthy breakfast. The whole grains found in cereals can be thought of as the "great regulators" because of their action on blood glucose, regularity, blood cholesterol and appetite. Eating breakfast cereals containing oats or less refined whole grains causes a more gradual rise in blood glucose and leaves you with a satisfied feeling. Wheat and oat bran (the outer layer of the whole kernel) add extra fibre to keep the digestive system healthy and to promote regularity. Oat bran and a low-fat diet help lower cholesterol levels. Flax seeds give our cereals a pleasant nutty flavour—and nutritionally much, much more. If ever a food was a "magic bullet," cereals may be it.

Use our recipes for **Crunchy Breakfast Oats** (page 42) and **Hot Seven-Grain Cereal** (page 48) to create your own grain-and-bran-rich "bulk mixes." They are easy to prepare in single servings. And all the ingredients can be found in bulk and health food stores so you can buy in just the amounts you need.

In addition, our breakfast menus use a variety of packaged, ready-to-eat whole grain and high-fibre cereals. Since everyone has his or her favourites, the words *"cereal of your choice"* in a menu refers you to Appendix 3, page 233, for a complete listing of cereals with serving sizes.

Breads and Muffins

Today there is an endless variety of breads available. When shopping for bread, the words "whole wheat" and "high-fibre" on the label suggest a wise choice. Multigrain breads may contain ingredients such as oats, oat bran, corn, barley, sunflower or sesame seeds yet still have white flour as their base. Read the list of ingredients on the wrapper and check the Nutrition Information panel for fibre content. Choose breads with at least 2 grams of fibre per serving.

Having a small scale on your kitchen counter lets you judge *how much* to eat since 1 STARCH CHOICE is equal to 1 ounce (30 grams) of bread containing 15 grams of carbohydrate. Most commercial muffins weigh at least 2 ounces (60 grams) and count as 2 STARCH CHOICES and the coffee shop variety often weigh 4 ounces (120 grams), with 50 or 60 grams of carbohydrate in each, and they are all high in fat as well. Homemade muffins can be made smaller and with a lower fat content than those you buy. They also freeze beautifully. There are several muffin recipes in our breakfast section alone (pages 37, 46, 49 and 54), all containing 20 grams of carbohydrate or less.

Margarine or Butter?

Our breakfast menus don't use much of either! A good-tasting bread or warm muffin needs little if any margarine or butter for flavour, thus reducing both fat and calories. Each breakfast menu contains 1 FATS & OILS CHOICE but often it's hidden in other foods.

Non-hydrogenated soft tub margarine is a better choice than butter because it contains less saturated fat. However, even margarine is fat that should be used in small amounts.

And if you still want more flavour, use a small amount of a low-sugar fruit spread.

Low-Sugar Fruit Spreads

We are always asked for recipes for low-sugar fruit spreads, so we offer **Light Raspberry Blueberry Spread** (page 33).

What about commercial fruit spreads? On your local grocery store shelf you'll find two kinds of fruit spreads, one labelled "No Sugar Added," the other "Light." Both contain fruit sweetened with a combination of concentrated fruit juice (usually white grape juice) and a non-nutritive sweetener such as sucralose or aspartame, or a form of sugar called sorbitol. The important difference between the two spreads is the *amount of carbohydrate per tablespoon (15 mL)*. Read the labels carefully. Each describes the amount of carbohydrate (read *sugars*) in 1 tbsp (15 mL) of spread. Before you use any fruit spread, we suggest you measure out one level tbsp (15 mL) so you can see how much it is. Remember that EXTRA doesn't mean "free."

Eggs, Milk and Yogurt

What to do about eggs? Current recommendations for a healthy person with no heart disease suggest reducing saturated fat and limiting cholesterol to no more than 300 mg per day. Since each egg yolk contains 2 grams of saturated fat and 215 milligrams of cholesterol, it seems wise to set a limit of three to four eggs per week. We suggest substituting two egg whites for one whole egg in some of our recipes.

We often think "eggs" when planning weekend or special breakfasts (see **Mushroom and Tomato Omelette** (page 47). However, **Oatmeal Pancakes** (page 34) with **Maple Yogurt Sauce** (page 35) or **Waffles with Fruit** (page 43) are special too.

All our breakfast menus include milk on cereal or as a recipe ingredient and there is always enough to put in tea or coffee. Low-fat milk means non-fat skim or 1%—your choice.

Yogurt is a great alternative to milk. Most people enjoy yogurt for its great taste, versatility and high nutritional value. Many who cannot tolerate milk find they can eat yogurt without a problem. Yogurt can be particularly useful for individuals who are recovering from flu or have been on antibiotics.

The Best Nutritional Bang

Since breakfast is such an important meal, make it a healthy start to your day. Include servings of fresh fruit along with whole grains such as cereals, whole wheat toast or healthy muffins for complex carbohydrate and fibre. Spread peanut butter on whole wheat toast for protein. Use a low-sugar fruit spread instead of margarine or butter. Add milk to the cereal for calcium. Such a breakfast gives us the nutrition we all need as well as limiting total fat, saturated fat and sodium. Breakfast already has you on the road to healthy eating!

breakfast menus

Each breakfast menu provides about 330 calories* and is based on:

2 STARCH CHOICES
1 FRUITS & VEGETABLES CHOICE
1 MILK (1%) CHOICE
1 PROTEIN CHOICE
1 FATS & OILS CHOICE

*319 calories with skim milk, 329 calories with 1% milk
46 grams carbohydrate

breakfast menu #1

1/2 small banana, sliced

1 shredded wheat biscuit
OR cereal of your choice (page 233)
with 1/2 cup (125 mL) low-fat milk

1 poached egg on 1 slice unbuttered whole wheat toast

coffee or tea

breakfast menu #2

1/2 grapefruit

1 small bagel (60 g), halved and toasted
with 2 tbsp (25 mL) light cream cheese

coffee or tea with milk

breakfast menu #3

1/2 cup (125 mL) blueberries

2/3 cup (150 mL) wheat bran flakes
OR cereal of your choice (page 233)
with 1/2 cup (125 mL) low-fat milk

1 egg, scrambled in nonstick pan in 1/2 tsp (2 mL) soft
margarine OR butter, with 1 slice unbuttered whole wheat toast

coffee or tea

breakfast menu #4

1/2 small banana, sliced

1 cup (250 mL) O-shaped toasted oat cereal
OR cereal of your choice (page 233)
with 1/2 cup (125 mL) low-fat milk

1 slice unbuttered whole wheat toast
with 1 tbsp (15 mL) peanut butter

coffee or tea

breakfast menu #5

2 stewed prunes with 1 tbsp (15 mL) juice

2/3 cup (150 mL) wheat bran flakes
OR cereal of your choice (page 233)
with 1/2 cup (125 mL) low-fat milk

1 boiled egg
1 slice whole wheat toast
1/2 tsp (2 mL) soft margarine OR butter
1 tbsp (15 mL) no-sugar-added fruit spread (page 19)

coffee or tea

breakfast menu #6

Bacon on a Kaiser
*1 slice (46 g) Canadian back bacon and 2 tomato slices in
1 toasted unbuttered Kaiser roll (60 g)*

coffee or tea with milk

breakfast menu #7

Bagel with Lox and Cream Cheese
1 medium bagel (90 g), halved
1 slice (20 g) smoked salmon
2 tbsp (25 mL) light cream cheese

sliced cucumbers and tomatoes

tea with lemon

breakfast menu #8

3/4 cup (175 mL) light cranberry cocktail

1 English muffin, halved and toasted,
with 2 slices (50 g) part-skim mozzarella cheese
1 tbsp (15 mL) no-sugar-added fruit spread (page 19)

coffee or tea with milk

breakfast menu #9

1 peach, sliced

2/3 cup (150 mL) wheat bran flakes
OR cereal of your choice (page 233)
with 1/2 cup (125 mL) low-fat milk

1 slice whole wheat toast
1 tbsp (15 mL) each: light peanut butter
and no-added-sugar fruit spread (page 19)

coffee or tea

breakfast menu #10

1/2 small banana, sliced

1/2 cup (125 mL) spoon-size shredded wheat cereal
OR cereal of your choice (page 233)
with 1/2 cup (125 mL) low-fat milk

1 soft-cooked egg
with 1 slice whole wheat toast

coffee or tea

breakfast menu #11

1/2 medium kiwi fruit, sliced and 1/2 cup (125 mL) sliced strawberries

1 soft-cooked egg
with 1 hot cross bun (65 g)
1 tbsp (15 mL) **Light Raspberry Blueberry Spread** (page 33)
OR 1 tbsp (15 mL) no-added-sugar fruit spread (page 19)

Café au Lait
1/2 cup (125 mL) each: hot strong coffee and hot low-fat milk

breakfast menu #12

A Greek Experience

1/2 orange

1 crusty roll (60 g) with 1 tsp (5 mL) soft margarine OR butter
1/4 cup (50 mL) low-fat plain yogurt and 1 tsp (5 mL) liquid honey

1 hard-cooked egg

coffee or tea with milk

breakfast menu #13

1/2 small orange

1 serving (1/6) **Oatmeal Pancakes** (page 34)
with 1/3 cup (75 mL) **Maple Yogurt Sauce** (page 35)

coffee or tea with milk

breakfast menu #14

1/2 pink grapefruit

Cooked Oat Bran Cereal
1/3 cup (75 mL) dry oat bran cereal made with 1 cup (250 mL) water
with 1/2 cup (125 mL) low-fat milk

1 **Banana Muffin** (page 37)
1 tsp (5 mL) soft margarine OR butter

coffee or tea

breakfast menu #15

2 slices **Cinnamon French Toast** (page 38)
with 1/2 cup (125 mL) warm unsweetened applesauce

coffee or tea with milk

breakfast menu #16

1/4 cantaloupe with lime wedge

Single-Serve Ham and Cheese Egg (page 39)

1 slice whole wheat toast
OR 1/2 toasted English muffin
1 tbsp (15 mL) no-sugar-added fruit spread (page 19)

coffee or tea with milk

breakfast menu #17

Strawberries 'n Dip (page 40)

1 cup (250 mL) O-shaped toasted oat cereal
OR cereal of your choice (page 233)
1/2 cup (125 mL) low-fat milk

1 slice toasted raisin bread
1/2 tsp (2 mL) soft margarine OR butter

coffee or tea

breakfast menu #18

1/2 grapefruit

Microwave Porridge for One (page 41)
with 1/2 cup (125 mL) low-fat milk
sweetener to taste

1 slice whole wheat toast,
1 tbsp (15 mL) peanut butter
and 1 tsp (5 mL) no-sugar-added fruit spread (page 19)

coffee or tea

breakfast menu #19

1/2 medium nectarine OR 1 peach, sliced

1/2 cup (125 mL) **Crunchy Breakfast Oats** (page 42)
with 1/2 cup (125 mL) low-fat milk

coffee or tea

breakfast menu #20

Waffles with Fruit (page 43)

coffee or tea with milk

breakfast menu #21

Peach-Berry Shake (page 44)

1/2 medium bagel (45 g)
with 1 tbsp (15 mL) crunchy peanut butter

coffee or tea with milk

breakfast menu #22

1/2 cup (125 mL) sliced strawberries OR 1/2 peach

1/2 cup (125 mL) spoon-size shredded wheat
OR cereal of your choice (page 233)
with 1/2 cup (125 mL) low-fat milk

1 **Double Bran Muffin** (page 46)
1/2 tsp (2 mL) soft margarine OR butter
1 tbsp (15 mL) no-sugar-added fruit spread (page 19)

coffee or tea

breakfast menu #23

Breakfast for Two

1 mandarin orange OR 1/2 grapefruit

1 serving (1/2) **Mushroom and Tomato Omelette** (page 47)

1 toasted English muffin OR 2 slices whole wheat toast
1 tbsp (15 mL) no-sugar-added fruit spread (page 19)

coffee or tea with milk

breakfast menu #24

1/2 pink grapefruit

1 serving **Hot Seven-Grain Cereal** (page 48)
with 1/2 cup (125 mL) low-fat milk
and granulated brown low-calorie sweetener

1/2 hot cross bun (30 g), toasted
1 tbsp (15 mL) peanut butter

coffee or tea

breakfast menu #25

1 kiwi fruit OR 1/3 mango

1 cup (250 mL) O-shaped toasted oat cereal
OR cereal of your choice (page 233)
with 1/2 cup (125 mL) low-fat milk

1 **Double Bran Muffin** (page 46)
1 tsp (5 mL) soft margarine OR butter

coffee or tea

breakfast menu #26

1 cup (250 mL) sliced strawberries
with 1/2 cup (125 mL) low-fat plain yogurt
and 1/2 cup (125 mL) high fibre wheat bran cereal
OR cereal of your choice (page 233)

1 **Raisin Bran Buttermilk Muffin** (page 49)
1 tsp (5 mL) soft margarine OR butter

coffee or tea with milk

breakfast menu #27

1/2 cup (125 mL) raspberries OR sliced strawberries
with 1/3 cup (75 mL) low-fat plain yogurt
and 1/3 cup (75 mL) high-fibre wheat bran cereal

1 **Ginger Bran Muffin** (page 50)
1 tsp (5 mL) soft margarine OR butter
1 tbsp (15 mL) no-added-sugar fruit spread (page 19)

coffee or tea

breakfast menu #28

1 serving (1/2) **Fruit Muesli** (page 51)

1 poached egg
with 1 slice whole wheat toast

coffee or tea with milk

breakfast menu #29

3 **Double-Bran Pancakes** (page 52)
with 1/2 cup (125 mL) sliced strawberries and
1/4 cup (50 mL) **Homemade Vanilla Yogurt** (page 53)
OR low-fat French vanilla yogurt, sweetened with aspartame

coffee or tea with milk

breakfast menu #30

1/2 cup (125 mL) sliced strawberries
with 1/4 cup (50 mL) low-fat French vanilla yogurt, sweetened with aspartame

1 shredded wheat biscuit
OR cereal of your choice (page 233)
with 1/2 cup (125 mL) low-fat milk

1 **Breakfast in a Muffin** (page 54)

coffee or tea

breakfast recipes index

breakfast recipes

breakfast menu # 8

Light Raspberry Blueberry Spread

The spread is so flavourful, it is hard to imagine it as low in carbohydrates!

ingredients

3 cups	raspberries (2 cups/500 mL crushed)	750 mL
2 cups	blueberries (1 cup/250 mL crushed)	500 mL
2 tbsp	lemon juice	25 mL
1 tsp	grated lemon rind	5 mL
1 cup	water	250 mL
1 box	(49 g) powdered fruit pectin crystals (see Tip)	1 box
2 tbsp	granulated sugar	25 mL
1 cup	granular low-calorie sweetener with sucralose (see Tip)	250 mL
1/4 tsp	ground nutmeg	1 mL

1 Crush raspberries and blueberries with a potato masher (you should have 3 cups/750 mL crushed fruit). Combine fruit, lemon juice and rind and water in medium stainless steel or enamel saucepan. Gradually stir in pectin.

2 Bring to full boil over medium-high heat, stirring constantly. Gradually stir in sugar, sweetener and nutmeg; return to boil and boil hard for 1 minute, stirring constantly.

3 Spoon spread into clean hot jars to within 1/2-inch (1 cm) of rim. Cover with tight-fitting lids. Label and refrigerate for up to three weeks or freeze for longer storage.

Makes 4 1/4 cups (1050 mL).

PREPARATION TIME:
about 15 minutes

COOKING TIME:
about 10 minutes

Each serving:
1 tbsp (15 mL)

1 EXTRA

3 g carbohydrate (0 g fibre)
0 g protein
0 g total fat
2 mg sodium
11 calories

KITCHEN TIP

Since this fruit spread recipe has the same Food Choice value, it can be used whenever a menu calls for a no-sugar-added variety.

Certo™ regular pectin has directions for making spreads without sugar. The low-sugar pectin from Bernardin is referred to as "no-sugar-needed" pectin and, as the name implies, can be made using no sugar or using some sugar and sweetener. Use either pectin when making this spread.

If you do not keep a bulk sweetener, then 10 packages of a low-calorie sweetener are a good replacement.

Use a potato masher to crush fruit rather than a food processor. The processor breaks down the texture of the fruit making it too mushy to retain its identity in the cooked spread.

PREPARATION TIME:
10 minutes

COOKING TIME:
about 4 minutes

Each serving:
3 pancakes (1/6 of recipe)

**2 STARCH CHOICES
1/2 FRUITS & VEGETABLES
CHOICE
1/2 PROTEIN CHOICE
1 FATS & OILS CHOICE**

37 g carbohydrate (2 g fibre)
9 g protein
6 g fat (2 g saturated fat)
54 mg sodium
240 calories

KITCHEN TIPS

For the best pancakes, don't over-mix—they'll become tough. Allow batter to sit for a few minutes before cooking.

Be sure to cook all the batter. Batter refrigerated for a day or so will yield thin, tough pancakes. Freeze extra cooked pancakes instead.

breakfast menu #13
Oatmeal Pancakes

Have your breakfast oatmeal in a pancake. Served with Maple Yogurt Sauce (see page 35), it makes a truly delicious breakfast.

1 1/4 cups	all purpose flour	300 mL
3/4 cup	quick-cooking rolled oats	175 mL
1 tbsp	granulated sugar	15 mL
1/2 tsp	ground cinnamon OR nutmeg	2 mL
1 1/2 cups	low-fat milk	375 mL
2	eggs, beaten	2
2/3 cup	unsweetened applesauce	150 mL
1 tbsp	canola oil	15 mL

1 In medium bowl, combine flour, rolled oats, sugar and cinnamon.

2 In second bowl, stir together milk, eggs and applesauce. Pour into dry ingredients; stir just until moistened (see Tip).

3 Heat oil in nonstick skillet over medium heat until hot. Pour batter with 1/4 cup (50 mL) measure into hot skillet; cook 2 minutes or until bubbles break on surface and underside is golden brown. Turn pancakes and cook just until bottom is lightly browned (see Tip).

Makes 6 servings, eighteen 3-inch (7.5 cm) pancakes.

breakfast menu #13
150-calorie snack menu #17

Maple Yogurt Sauce

Maple Yogurt Sauce is the perfect accompaniment to **Oatmeal Pancakes** (see page 34). It only tastes rich, but is really very low calorie.

2 cups	low-fat plain yogurt	500 mL
4 tsp	granulated brown low-calorie sweetener (see Tip)	20 mL
1/2 tsp	maple extract	2 mL
1/2 tsp	ground cinnamon	2 mL

1 In bowl, combine yogurt, sweetener, maple extract and cinnamon.

2 Refrigerate until ready to serve.

Makes 6 servings, 2 cups (500 mL) sauce.

PREPARATION TIME:
5 minutes

Each serving:
1/3 cup (75 mL)

1 MILK 2% CHOICE

6 g carbohydrate (0 g fibre)
4 g protein
1 g fat (1 g saturated fat)
63 mg sodium
52 calories

KITCHEN TIP

Liquid cyclamate sweetener (1 1/4 tsp/ 6 mL) can replace granulated sweetener in this recipe.

PREPARATION TIME:
10 minutes

KITCHEN TIP

Stored in the refrigerator, **Multimix** keeps for two months. For other **Multimix** recipes, see pages 37, 139, 183, 185, 191 and 217.

breakfast menu #13

150-calorie snack menus #14, #16, #31
dinner menu #15
special occasions menu #4

Multimix

Keep this handy mix stored in the refrigerator for fast preparation of pancakes, muffins, scones and tea biscuits.

3 cups	all purpose flour	750 mL
2 cups	whole wheat flour	500 mL
3 tbsp	baking powder	45 mL
1 cup	soft margarine OR butter	250 mL

1 In large bowl, combine flours and baking powder. Mix in margarine until mixture resembles coarse crumbs or blend the mixture in a food processor bowl.

2 Store in refrigerator in airtight container (see Tip).

Makes about 8 cups (2 L).

breakfast menu #14

150-calorie snack menu #27

Banana Muffins

Warm Banana Muffins are wonderfully satisfying at breakfast, or pack them as a snack with your lunch.

2 cups	**Multimix** (see page 36)	500 mL
2 tbsp	granulated sugar	25 mL
1/2 tsp	baking soda	2 mL
2/3 cup	mashed banana (1 1/2 small)	150 mL
1/2 cup	buttermilk or sour milk (see Tip)	125 mL
1	egg, beaten	1
1 tsp	vanilla extract	5 mL

1 In medium bowl, combine **Multimix**, sugar and baking soda.

2 In small bowl, stir together banana, buttermilk, egg and vanilla. Pour into dry ingredients; stir just until combined.

3 Spoon batter evenly into 12 nonstick or paper-lined medium muffin cups. Bake in 400°F (200°C) oven for 20 minutes or until firm to the touch.

Makes 12 medium muffins.

PREPARATION TIME:
10 minutes

COOKING TIME:
20 minutes

Each serving:
1 muffin

1 STARCH CHOICE
1 FATS & OILS CHOICE

17 g carbohydrate (**1 g fibre**)
3 g protein
6 g total fat (1 g saturated fat)
120 mg sodium
125 calories

KITCHEN TIP

To sour milk, stir 1 tsp (5 mL) lemon juice or vinegar into 1/2 cup (125 mL) milk; let stand for a few minutes.

PREPARATION TIME:
about 10 minutes

COOKING TIME:
5 minutes

Each serving:
2 slices

2 STARCH CHOICES
1/2 MILK 2% CHOICE
1 PROTEIN CHOICE
1 FATS & OILS CHOICE

33 g carbohydrate (1 g fibre)
14 g protein
10 g total fat (3 g saturated fat)
939 mg sodium
288 calories

KITCHEN TIP

Make extra French toast. Allow to cool completely before wrapping each slice separately for the freezer.

breakfast menu #15
Cinnamon French Toast

Ground cinnamon provides the homey aroma and flavor, and honey the sweetness in this version of classic French toast. Ideal for a leisurely weekend breakfast.

French Toast

1/3 cup	low-fat milk	75 mL
1	egg, lightly beaten	1
1/2 tsp	ground cinnamon	2 mL
1/4 tsp	salt	1 mL
1/4 tsp	vanilla extract	1 mL
2	slices white OR whole wheat bread	2
1/2 tsp	soft margarine OR butter	2 mL

1 In shallow pie plate, combine milk, egg, cinnamon, salt and vanilla extract. Dip each bread slice into egg mixture, coating each side well.

2 In large nonstick skillet, melt margarine over medium heat. Cook bread for 2 minutes each side or until golden brown.

Makes 1 serving.

OVEN PREPARATION:
Melt margarine on nonstick baking pan in 400°F (200°C) oven. Place dipped bread slices on pan. Bake for about 10 minutes per side. This makes a crisper French toast.

breakfast menu #16

Single-Serve Ham and Cheese Egg

A small amount of ham added to an egg goes a long way. This one-serving recipe tastes great any time of day!

2 tbsp	finely chopped ham	25 mL
1 tbsp	chopped celery	15 mL
1 tbsp	chopped onion	15 mL
1/2 tsp	soft margarine OR butter	2 mL
1	egg, beaten OR 2 egg whites	1
Pinch	each: pepper and paprika	Pinch
1 tbsp	shredded mozzarella cheese	15 mL
1/2	English muffin, toasted OR 1 slice whole wheat bread	1/2

1 In small custard cup, combine ham, celery, onion and margarine. Microwave, uncovered, on High (100%) for 2 minutes.

2 Stir in egg and seasonings. Microwave on Medium-High (70%) for 45 seconds; stir once.

3 Top with shredded cheese; let stand for about 1 minute to allow cheese to melt.

4 Serve on a toasted English muffin half or whole wheat toast.

Makes 1 serving.

PREPARATION TIME:
5 minutes

COOKING TIME:
about 3 minutes

Each serving:
1 egg on 1/2 English muffin

1 STARCH CHOICE
1 1/2 PROTEIN CHOICES
1 FATS & OILS CHOICE

15 g carbohydrate (**1 g fibre**)
14 g protein
10 g total fat (3 g saturated fat)
523 mg sodium
208 calories

PREPARATION TIME:
5 minutes

Each serving:
10 strawberries and 1/4 cup (50 mL) dip

1 FRUITS & VEGETABLES CHOICE
1/2 MILK SKIM CHOICE
1 FATS & OILS CHOICE

15 g carbohydrate (3 g fibre)
3 g protein
5 g total fat (3 g saturated fat)
22 mg sodium
115 calories

breakfast menu #17
Strawberries 'n Dip

We are indeed fortunate to be able to buy fresh strawberries throughout much of the year. And an easy dip for a year-round breakfast treat.

10	fresh ripe strawberries	10
1/4 cup	light sour cream	50 mL
1/4 tsp	vanilla OR almond extract	1 mL
	Sweetener to taste	

1 Arrange strawberries on a serving plate.

2 In a small bowl, stir together sour cream, vanilla extract and sweetener to taste.

3 Serve as a dip with strawberries.

Makes 1/4 cup (50 mL) dip.

breakfast menu #18

Microwave Porridge for One

Kick-start your day with this cooked hot cereal, rich in soluble fibre.

1/2 cup	water	125 mL
1/4 cup	quick-cooking rolled oats	50 mL
1/4 tsp	vanilla or maple extract	1 mL

For a double serving, use 1 cup (250 mL) water and 1/2 cup (125 mL) rolled oats.

1 In microwave-safe serving bowl, combine water, rolled oats and vanilla extract. Microwave, uncovered, on High (100%) for 1 1/2 to 2 minutes; stir once. Let stand for 1 to 2 minutes or until desired consistency. Stir and serve.

2 For a thinner porridge, add 1 to 2 tbsp (15 to 25 mL) more water.

Makes 1 serving.

Stovetop Porridge for the Family:

In saucepan, combine 1 cup (250 mL) rolled oats and 2 cups (500 mL) water. Cook on medium heat for 5 minutes or until thickened; stir occasionally. Cover, remove from heat; let stand a few minutes before serving.

Makes 4 servings, 2 cups (500 mL).

PREPARATION TIME:
under 5 minutes

COOKING TIME:
1 1/2 to 2 minutes

Each serving:
1/2 cup (125 mL)

1 STARCH CHOICE

14 g carbohydrate (2 g fibre)
3 g protein
1 g total fat (0 g saturated fat)
4 mg sodium
79 calories

PREPARATION TIME:
10 minutes

COOKING TIME:
8 to 10 minutes

Each serving:
1/2 cup (125 mL)

1 STARCH CHOICE
1 FRUITS & VEGETABLES CHOICE
1/2 PROTEIN CHOICE
2 FATS & OILS CHOICES

31 g carbohydrate (5 g fibre)
8 g protein
11 g total fat (2 g saturated fat)
32 mg sodium
240 calories

breakfast menu #19
Crunchy Breakfast Oats

More commonly referred to as granola, in this version the fat and sugar, but not the fibre, have been reduced.

1 1/2 cups	quick-cooking rolled oats	375 mL
1/2 cup	natural bran	125 mL
1/4 cup	wheat germ	50 mL
3 tbsp	chopped almonds	45 mL
2 tbsp	liquid honey	25 mL
2 tbsp	soft margarine OR butter	25 mL
2 tbsp	water	25 mL
1/4 cup	skim milk powder	50 mL
1/4 cup	raisins	50 mL
1/4 cup	unsweetened coconut	50 mL
1/4 cup	sunflower seeds	50 mL
1 tsp	ground cinnamon	5 mL

1 In large bowl, combine oats, bran, wheat germ and almonds.

2 In saucepan, heat honey, margarine and water until hot. Stir into oat mixture. Spread on baking pan.

3 Bake in 350°F (180°C) oven for 10 minutes or until lightly toasted; stir once. Let cool completely.

4 Stir in skim milk powder, raisins, coconut, sunflower seeds and cinnamon. Store in tightly sealed container.

Makes 7 servings, 3 1/2 cups (875 mL).

breakfast menu #20

Waffles with Fruit

Waffles served with a variety of fruits make a colourful, tasty and very nutritious breakfast.

2	frozen multigrain waffles	2
1/4 cup	low-fat cottage cheese	50 mL
2 tbsp	raspberries	25 mL
1/4	small banana, sliced	1/4
1/4	slice fresh pineapple, cubed	1/4
1/4	small orange, sliced	1/4
2 tbsp	low-fat (1%) plain yogurt	25 mL
Pinch	ground cinnamon	Pinch

1 Toast waffles until golden brown. Top with cottage cheese. Arrange raspberries, banana, pineapple and orange on plate. Top with yogurt and a sprinkle of cinnamon.

Makes 1 serving.

PREPARATION TIME:
10 minutes

COOKING TIME:
1 minute in toaster

Each serving:
1 recipe

2 STARCH CHOICES
1 1/2 FRUITS & VEGETABLES CHOICES
1 1/2 PROTEIN CHOICES
1 FATS & OILS CHOICE

48 g carbohydrate (4 g fibre)
15 g protein
9 g total fat (0 g saturated fat)
656 mg sodium
309 calories

PREPARATION TIME:
5 minutes

Each serving:
1 tall glass

1 FRUITS & VEGETABLES CHOICE
1 1/2 MILK 1% CHOICES

22 g carbohydrate (**3 g fibre**)
8 g protein
2 g total fat (1 g saturated fat)
105 mg sodium
130 calories

Peach-Berry Shake

Here's a tasty, refreshing beverage that's also good for you. And being a single serving, it's ideal whenever you are on your own. Or it can be doubled for two people.

1/2 cup	low-fat milk	125 mL
1/2 cup	raspberries or sliced strawberries	125 mL
1/4 cup	low-fat (1%) plain yogurt	50 mL
1/2	small ripe peach, peeled	1/2
2	ice cubes	2
	Sweetener to taste	

1 In blender container or food processor bowl, combine milk, raspberries, yogurt, peach and ice cubes.

2 Blend at high speed until smooth. Add sweetener to taste. Pour into a glass and enjoy.

Makes 1 serving.

breakfast menus #22, #25, #29
300-calorie snack menus #15, #16

Make-Ahead Double Bran Muffin Batter

This excellent refrigerator muffin batter allows one to quickly make small batches of fresh muffins as needed (see page 46). Or if you prefer to have pancakes, see our recipe on page 52 using this same basic batter. The refrigerated batter keeps up to two weeks.

Basic Muffin Batter

1 cup	boiling water	250 mL
1 1/2 cups	high-fibre wheat bran cereal (see Tip)	375 mL
2 cups	buttermilk	500 mL
1/2 cup	canola oil	125 mL
1/3 cup	molasses	75 mL
2	eggs, beaten OR 4 egg whites	2
1 tsp	vanilla extract	5 mL
1 cup	whole wheat flour	250 mL
1 cup	all purpose flour	250 mL
1 cup	oat bran	250 mL
1/2 cup	granular low-calorie sweetener with sucralose	125 mL
1/3 cup	granulated sugar	75 mL
1 tbsp	baking soda	15 mL

PREPARATION TIME: 15 minutes

1 In bowl, stir boiling water into wheat bran cereal (see Tip); let cool for 10 minutes. Stir in buttermilk, oil, molasses, eggs and vanilla.

2 In large bowl, combine flours, oat bran, sweetener, sugar and baking soda. Add buttermilk mixture; stir just until moistened. Place in large tightly sealed container and refrigerate for up to two weeks.

Makes 6 cups (1.5 L) batter.

PREPARATION TIME:
5 minutes

COOKING TIME:
20 minutes

Each serving:
1 muffin

1/2 STARCH CHOICE
1 SUGARS CHOICE
1/2 PROTEIN CHOICE
1 FATS & OILS CHOICE

20 g carbohydrate (3 g fibre)
4 g protein
6 g total fat (1 g saturated fat)
214 mg sodium
140 calories

breakfast menus #22, #25

150-calorie snack menu #23

Double Bran Muffins

To make 6 muffins using the very handy refrigerator **Make-Ahead Double Bran Muffin Batter** (page 45), follow the directions below for hot and satisfying muffins.

| 1 1/2 cups | **Make-Ahead Double Bran Muffin Batter** | 375 mL |

1 Spoon batter evenly into 6 nonstick or paper-lined medium muffin cups, filling 3/4 full.

2 Bake in 375°F (190°C) oven for 20 minutes or until firm to the touch.

Makes 6 medium muffins.

breakfast menu #23

Mushroom and Tomato Omelette

An omelette has to be the most elegant and satisfying way to serve breakfast eggs. It becomes the star of any leisurely weekend breakfast. This simple recipe serves two, but can be halved for a single serving.

1 tsp	soft margarine OR butter	5 mL
3	sliced mushrooms	3
1	sliced green onion	1
1/2	medium tomato, chopped	1/2
2	eggs, beaten	2
Pinch	each: salt and pepper	Pinch

1 In nonstick skillet, melt margarine on medium-high heat. Add mushrooms, onion and tomato; cook until softened, stirring frequently.

2 Add eggs, salt and pepper. Cook on medium heat for 2 minutes or until eggs are set.

Makes 2 servings.

PREPARATION TIME:
10 minutes

COOKING TIME:
5 minutes

Each serving:
1/2 omelette

1 PROTEIN CHOICE
1 FATS & OILS CHOICE
1 EXTRA

3 g carbohydrate (1 g fibre)
7 g protein
7 g total fat (2 g saturated fat)
321 mg sodium
105 calories

PREPARATION TIME:
for dry mix, 5 minutes

COOKING TIME:
for 1 serving, 5 minutes

Each serving:
1/4 cup (50 mL) of dry mix
(3/4 cup/175 mL cooked)

1 STARCH CHOICE
1/2 PROTEIN CHOICE

21 g carbohydrate (3 g fibre)
4 g protein
1 g total fat (0 g saturated fat)
3 mg sodium
108 calories

KITCHEN TIPS

Look for a combination of cracked wheat, cracked rye and whole flax when choosing a three-grain cereal. Flax seeds contain several essential nutrients, including calcium, iron, phosphorus and vitamin E and are a rich source of omega-3 fatty acids.

Wheat flakes are whole wheat berries that have been flattened between rollers. They resemble rolled oats and can be used in much the same way.

breakfast menu #24
Hot Seven-Grain Cereal

Start the day off right with seven healthy grains in your cereal bowl. One serving of this hot cooked cereal contains a moderate source of fibre and is a good source of iron.

Dry Cereal Mix

1 cup	large-flake rolled oats	250 mL
1 cup	three-grain cereal (see Tip)	250 mL
1 cup	rolled wheat flakes (see Tip)	250 mL
1/2 cup	oat bran	125 mL
1/2 cup	Cream of Wheat	125 mL

1 Combine rolled oats, three-grain cereal, whole wheat flakes, oat bran and cream of wheat. Store in tightly sealed container.

Makes 16 servings, 4 cups (1 L).

For Single Serving

Microwave: In microwave-safe serving bowl, combine 1/4 cup (50 mL) dry cereal mix and 3/4 cup (175 mL) water. Microwave, uncovered, on High (100%) for 2 minutes; stir. Microwave on Low (30%) for 3 minutes. Let stand for 2 minutes. Stir and serve.

Stovetop: In saucepan, combine ingredients (see above). Bring to boil, reduce heat to medium-low; cook 5 minutes or until desired consistency, stirring occasionally. Cover and remove from heat; let stand a few minutes. Stir and serve.

breakfast menu #26

150-calorie snack menu #25
300-calorie snack menu #10

Raisin Bran Buttermilk Muffins

High-fibre muffins are always a breakfast hit. This is an extremely reliable recipe with several variations.

1 1/2 cups	buttermilk (see Tip)	375 mL
1 1/2 cups	high-fibre wheat bran cereal (see Tip)	375 mL
1	egg, beaten	1
3 tbsp	canola oil	45 mL
1 tsp	vanilla extract	5 mL
1 cup	whole wheat flour	250 mL
2 tbsp	granulated sugar	25 mL
2 tsp	baking powder	10 mL
1/2 tsp	baking soda	2 mL
2 tbsp	raisins, chopped	25 mL

1 In bowl, stir buttermilk into cereal; let stand for 5 minutes or until cereal is softened. Beat in egg, oil and vanilla extract.

2 In large bowl, combine flour, sugar, baking powder, baking soda and raisins. Add buttermilk mixture; stir just until combined.

3 Spoon batter evenly into 12 nonstick or paper-lined medium muffin cups. Bake in 400°F (200°C) oven for 20 minutes or until firm to the touch.

Makes 12 medium muffins.

PREPARATION TIME:
15 minutes

COOKING TIME:
20 minutes

Each serving:
1 muffin

Muffin Variations
Replace raisins with:
2 tbsp (25 mL) chopped dried apricots (4 halves) OR

1/2 cup (125 mL) fresh or frozen blueberries and 1/2 tsp (2 mL) ground cinnamon OR

1/2 cup (125 mL) chopped apple (1/2 medium apple) and 1/2 tsp (2 mL) ground nutmeg

1 STARCH CHOICE
1 FATS & OILS CHOICE

20 g carbohydrate (4 g fibre)
4 g protein
5 g total fat (1 g saturated fat)
207 mg sodium
123 calories

KITCHEN TIPS

If you don't have buttermilk, stir 4 tsp (20 mL) vinegar or lemon juice into 1 1/2 cups (375 mL) milk; let stand for 5 minutes.

All Bran and Bran Cereal are examples of high-fibre wheat bran cereals.

PREPARATION TIME:
15 minutes

COOKING TIME:
about 18 minutes

Each serving:
1 muffin

1 STARCH CHOICE
1/2 SUGARS CHOICE
1 FATS & OILS CHOICE

23 g carbohydrate (4 g fibre)
4 g protein
5 g total fat (1 g saturated fat)
124 mg sodium
140 calories

KITCHEN TIP

Natural wheat bran is the outer layer of the wheat kernel that is removed during milling. Bran is a good source of fibre, calcium and phosphorus and is found in cereals and baked goods. It can be purchased at health food stores and supermarkets.

breakfast menu #27
special occasions menu #3

Ginger Bran Muffins

Ginger gives a flavour lift to the bran of these hearty muffins. Natural wheat bran, the outer covering of the wheat berry, has very little nutritional value but plenty of fibre. Look for it in the cereal section of the supermarket or in health food stores.

1 1/2 cups	natural wheat bran (see Tip)	375 mL
1 cup	all purpose flour	250 mL
1 cup	whole wheat flour	250 mL
2 tbsp	granular low-calorie sweetener with sucralose	25 mL
1 tbsp	granulated sugar	15 mL
2 tsp	ground ginger	10 mL
1 tsp	each: baking powder and baking soda	5 mL
2 cups	buttermilk	500 mL
1/3 cup	fancy molasses	75 mL
1/4 cup	canola oil	50 mL
1	egg, beaten	1
3 tbsp	chopped candied ginger	45 mL

1 In large bowl, combine bran, flours, sweetener, sugar, ginger, baking powder and baking soda.

2 In medium bowl, stir together buttermilk, molasses, oil and egg. Pour into dry ingredients; stir just until moistened. Stir in candied ginger.

3 Spoon batter evenly in 16 nonstick or paper-lined medium muffin cups. Bake in 375°F (190°C) oven for 20 minutes or until firm to touch.

Makes 16 medium muffins.

breakfast menu #28
Fruit Muesli

A popular European breakfast, this version puts the orange juice, fruit and rolled oats together for an easy start to the day.

1/2 cup	large-flake rolled oats	125 mL
1/4 cup	orange juice (see Tip)	50 mL
1 tbsp	chopped raisins	15 mL
1 tsp	liquid honey	5 mL
1/2 tsp	vanilla extract	2 mL
2	medium strawberries, sliced	2
1/4 cup	mashed bananas	50 mL
1/3 cup	low-fat (1%) plain yogurt OR low-fat milk (see Tip)	75 mL

1 In medium bowl, combine rolled oats, orange juice, raisins, honey and vanilla. Cover and refrigerate overnight (see Tip).

2 In morning, stir in strawberries, banana and yogurt. Spoon into cereal bowls and serve.

Makes 2 servings.

PREPARATION TIME:
10 minutes

CHILL:
overnight

Each serving:
1/2 recipe

1 STARCH CHOICE
1/2 PROTEIN CHOICE
1/2 FATS & OILS CHOICE

37 g carbohydrate (**4 g fibre**)
6 g protein
2 g total fat (0 g saturated fat)
31 mg sodium
187 calories

KITCHEN TIPS

Keep a can of concentrated orange juice in your freezer. 1 tbsp (15 mL) frozen concentrate with 3 tbsp (45 mL) water gives you the 1/4 cup (50 mL) orange juice needed in this recipe. Keep the rest frozen.

Muesli mixed with low-fat milk and refrigerated overnight, has the consistency of cooked cereal.

PREPARATION TIME:
3 minutes

COOKING TIME:
under 5 minutes

Each serving:
3 pancakes

1 1/2 STARCH CHOICES
1 SUGARS CHOICE
1/2 PROTEIN CHOICE
2 FATS & OILS CHOICES

40 g carbohydrate (**6 g fibre**)
7 g protein
12 g total fat (1 g saturated fat)
407 mg sodium
280 calories

breakfast menu #29
Double Bran Pancakes

To quickly make one serving of pancakes using the handy **Make-Ahead Double Bran Muffin Batter** (page 45), follow these easy directions below.

1/2 cup	**Make-Ahead Double Bran Muffin Batter**	125 mL
2 tbsp	water	25 mL

1 In small bowl, stir together batter and water. Heat non-stick skillet over medium (see Tip). Spray with non-stick cooking spray. Drop batter by spoonfuls into hot skillet to make 3 thin pancakes.

2 Cook pancakes for about 3 minutes or until bubbles break on surface; turn and cook second side until golden. Since these pancakes darken quickly, watch that the heat remains at medium.

Makes 3 pancakes.

breakfast menu #29

Homemade Vanilla Yogurt

Want a change from plain yogurt but don't want to buy another large container of a flavoured one? Just add a flavouring and sweetener to your plain yogurt. Try vanilla or one of our suggested variations.

1 cup	low-fat (1%) plain yogurt	250 mL
1/2–1 tsp	vanilla extract	2–5 mL
	Low-calorie sweetener (see Tip)	

1 In small bowl, stir together yogurt, vanilla and sweetener. Cover and refrigerate a short time to allow flavours to develop.

Makes 1 cup (250 mL).

PREPARATION TIME:
5 minutes

CHILL:
as long as yogurt keeps fresh (see expiry on original container)

Each serving:
1/4 cup (50 mL)

1/2 MILK 1% CHOICE

5 g carbohydrate (0 g fibre)
3 g protein
0 g total fat
44 mg sodium
34 calories

Variations
Maple or Rum Nutmeg: add maple or rum extract and ground nutmeg. Or add lemon, orange or almond extract (without the nutmeg).

KITCHEN TIP

Taste after adding the extract and before any sweetener. The flavour may be sweet enough. If still too tart, add sweetener to taste.

PREPARATION TIME:
15 minutes

COOKING TIME:
about 20 minutes

Each serving:
1 muffin

1 STARCH CHOICE
1/2 SUGARS CHOICE
1/2 PROTEIN CHOICE
1 FATS & OILS CHOICE

20 g carbohydrate (1 g fibre)
6 g protein
7 g total fat (1 g saturated fat)
194 mg sodium
162 calories

breakfast menu #30
Breakfast in a Muffin

Bacon, Cheddar cheese and egg make these muffins a hearty breakfast.

2	slices bacon-style turkey, cooked	2
1 3/4 cups	all purpose flour	425 mL
2/3 cup	oat bran	150 mL
1/4 cup	granulated sugar	50 mL
2 tbsp	granular low-calorie sweetener with sucralose	25 mL
2 1/2 tsp	baking powder	12 mL
1/2 tsp	baking soda	2 mL
1/4 tsp	each: dried oregano and paprika	1 mL
1 cup	shredded light Cheddar cheese	250 mL
2	green onions, thinly sliced	2
1 1/4 cups	buttermilk	300 mL
1/4 cup	canola oil	50 mL
1	egg OR 2 egg whites, slightly beaten	1

1 Crumble cooked bacon into small pieces. In large bowl, combine bacon, flour, oat bran, sugar, sweetener, baking powder, baking soda, oregano, paprika, cheese and onions.

2 In second bowl, combine buttermilk, oil and egg. Pour into dry ingredients; stir just until combined.

3 Divide batter evenly between 12 nonstick or paper-lined medium muffin cups, filling 2/3 full. Bake in 400°F (200°C) oven for 20 minutes or until firm to the touch.

Makes 12 medium muffins.

lunch

What's for Lunch?

Soup, a sandwich and a salad are old standbys. And rightly so. Each makes an easily prepared nutritious meal to satisfy midday hunger pangs. Soups and sandwiches can be served hot in the winter and cold in the summer. But the same old selections day after day become oh so dull. Our lunch recipes and menus offer new twists on old favourites as well as some nifty new lunch ideas.

Lunch is a marvelous time to stock up on nutrition. Soup, depending on the variety, can have fibre and protein from barley, lentils and beans, protein from meat, and vitamins and minerals from vegetables. Sandwiches made with whole wheat breads are full of fibre to say nothing of the fibre, protein, vitamins and minerals in the fillings. And a low-fat salad is really just a tasty medley of fibre, vitamins and minerals finished off with protein from any added meat or cheese.

Soups

We think soup is one of the most perfect foods. It's economical, easy to make, gets better with each reheating and tends to be low in fat. A pot of soup simmering on the stove gives warmth and comfort on a cold blustery winter day. A freezer filled with an assortment of frozen portions means that a nourishing lunch is not far away.

This chapter offers several quite different hot soups. **Hearty Vegetable Barley Soup** (page 93) and **Curried Vegetable and Split Pea Soup** (page 73) are all filled with plain old-fashioned goodness, as well as slowly digested low glycemic carbohydrates. When time is limited, either **Baked Bean Soup** (page 87) or **Soup 'n Sandwich in a Bowl** (page 85) make a fast, simple and nutritious lunch.

Soups are best made with **Homemade Chicken Broth** and we think our recipe is a good one (see page 91). Whenever you see a reference to chicken broth in a recipe, think homemade! Your soup will taste better and you control the salt level—an important consideration if you have been advised to limit sodium intake. See page 7 for more about salt and hypertension.

If you are cooking for one or two, you may wonder if it's worth the bother to make your own soups. We say it is. All our soup recipes freeze well for up to two months.

Sandwiches

Sandwiches are an ideal lunch for one- and two-person households. Each is a custom creation of just the right amount for a person to eat at one sitting.

Bread in a sandwich does more than just hold the filling; it adds flavour, texture and variety to the total sandwich. Breads come in all shapes and sizes, as do buns, bagels, baguettes, pita breads and wraps (flour tortillas). And they all come in whole wheat and multigrain versions. Each gives the filling a different taste. And do we have fillings! How about our slant on traditional **Tuna Sandwich Filling** (page 69) and **Egg Dill Sandwich Filling** (page 74), or try **Salmon Pecan Sandwich Filling** (page 86) for a heart-healthy lunch rich in omega-3 fatty acids.

But the variety of sizes in bread products can create a problem for those with diabetes. For example, how big a bagel or how large a slice of bread did we mean in a certain menu, when bagels and breads come in such a variety of sizes? To deal with this, we have assigned weights to bread products used in our menus and recipes, remembering that a 30 gram roll or slice of bread contains 15 grams of carbohydrate, equal to 1 STARCH CHOICE.

A little extra touch, like toasting the bun or the bread for a sandwich, makes a great sandwich taste even better.

Salads

How to make salads more interesting? There are so many nifty things you can do to a salad that it has become one of our favourite topics! It's a challenge that we wish some restaurants would meet. After all, a boring salad makes a boring lunch.

The Greens

The profusion of salad greens now readily available gives us a riot of exciting choices—and they can all be used generously in a diabetes meal plan.

One green often overlooked is Belgian endive. It has a pleasantly bitter flavour. Trim off the bottom and separate the leaves to use with other greens or to stuff with a filling. Another is watercress, a great complement to other greens or a background to tomatoes. A member of the mustard family, watercress is very peppery and intense. Look for it in bunches in the produce section.

How Do I Make a Salad Work?

1. Wash leafy greens and use a salad spinner to dry. They keep fresher if wrapped in paper or cloth towelling and stored in a tightly sealed plastic container in the refrigerator. Or use one of the new ventilated plastic storage bags. Lettuce and spinach purchased in airtight packaging should be refrigerated as is.

2. Tear greens, don't chop, for crisper salads.

3. The darker the greens, the more nutrients.

4. Keep some dinner vegetables raw and use in a green salad. Small broccoli and cauliflower florets, shredded carrots and chopped bok choy are other candidates. Some of our recipes add fresh fruit to a salad for a refreshing change—see **Cabbage Waldorf Salad** (page 72) and **Fruit Plate with Ricotta Cheese** (page 76). Or eat your salad in a pita—see **Greek Salad in a Pita** (page 92).

5. Use fresh herbs such as basil, dill, oregano or tarragon in salads.

6. Toss greens with the dressing at the last minute.

The Dressing

A salad dressing can make or break a salad. The ideal dressing lightly coats your salad, complements the flavours and textures of the ingredients and highlights the key flavours. A heavy or boring dressing insults fresh greens.

On top of all this, the dressing should be low in fat. Surveys show salad dressings to be one of the chief sources of added fat in the Canadian diet. Choose one of the many commercial low-fat dressings now available. Another approach is to make your own—then you know what's in it. Try one of our homemade low-fat dressings like **Herb Vinaigrette** (page 128) or **Favourite Caesar Salad Dressing** (page 133).

Here are some tips for lowering fat in dressings:

- Lighten mayonnaise with lemon juice, vinegar, low-fat plain yogurt or milk.
- Choose the light reduced-fat mayonnaises and salad dressings.
- Mix salsa with yogurt to make a super-light tasty dressing.
- When eating out, ask for a lower-fat dressing on the side and add just what you need.

What Are Specialty Vinegars?

Specialty vinegars may be:

- Flavoured, such as raspberry, garlic, or blueberry vinegars,
- Herb-steeped, such as tarragon, basil, or thyme vinegars,
- Fermented, such as rice, or red or white wine vinegars OR
- The royalty of all vinegars, balsamic.

Are You Ready for an Oil Change?

Predominately unsaturated oils (see Appendix 1, page 223) are the healthiest oils for dressings. Canola is the most unsaturated vegetable oil and it is one of the cheapest and most widely available in Canada. Safflower, sunflower, corn and olive oils (in descending order) are almost as unsaturated. However, all vegetable oils are fats and should be used sparingly.

Specialty oils like sesame, hazelnut and walnut deliver fantastic flavours, allowing you to use a lesser quantity, which is good since they are rather expensive. After opening, they will keep fresh in a refrigerator for about a year.

Desserts

Desserts give a nice finish to lunch. Our lunchtime desserts are mainly fruit, served raw, or cooked in simple recipes like **Microwave Applesauce** (page 75). Fruit delivers the sweetness we would expect from a dessert but with relatively few calories and lots of fibre, minerals and vitamins. And if you don't have the fruit on hand suggested in a menu, check Appendix 2, page 227, for other fruit choices.

lunch menus

Each lunch menu provides about 430 calories* and is based on:

2 STARCH CHOICES
2 FRUITS & VEGETABLES CHOICES
1 MILK (1%) CHOICE
2 PROTEIN CHOICES
1 FATS & OILS CHOICE
1 EXTRA

*419 calories with skim milk, 429 calories with 1% milk
56 grams carbohydrate

lunch menu #1

1 cup (250 mL) cream of celery soup made with low-fat milk

1/4 cup (50 mL) salmon with lettuce
on 1/2 toasted bagel (45 g)

1/2 cup (125 mL) unsweetened applesauce
2 arrowroot cookies

lunch menu #2

Cheese and Pineapple Melt
*2 slices (50 g) processed cheese
melted over 2 slices canned pineapple
on 2 toasted English muffin halves (60 g)*

1/2 cup (125 mL) low-fat milk

lunch menu #3

2 slices (60 g) lean cooked ham
mustard, lettuce and 2 tsp (10 mL) light mayonnaise
on 2 slices multigrain bread (60 g)

1 cup (250 mL) low-fat fruit yogurt

lunch menu #4
Pub Lunch

microwave 1 medium (190 g) potato; top with sliced green onion and 1/2 cup (125 mL) shredded light Cheddar cheese

1 mandarin orange OR fruit of your choice (page 227)

1/2 cup (125 mL) low-fat milk

lunch menu #5

1 cup (250 mL) split pea soup

1 wedge (25 g) light Cheddar cheese
4 whole wheat soda crackers

1 medium apple OR fruit of your choice (page 227)

1/2 cup (125 mL) low-fat milk

lunch menu #6

1/2 can tomato soup made with low-fat milk

Grilled Cheese Sandwich
2 slices whole wheat toast with 1 slice (25 g) processed cheese heated in nonstick pan until cheese melts

1 small carrot, cut into sticks

lunch menu #7

Peanut Butter and Banana Sandwich
2 slices raisin bread spread with 2 tbsp (25 mL) light peanut butter and 1/2 small banana, sliced

1 cup (250 mL) low-fat milk

lunch menu #8

1/4 cup (50 mL) **Tuna Sandwich Filling** (page 69) on 2 slices whole wheat bread with lettuce

1 serving (1/2) **Blender Yogurt Fruit Shake** (page 69)

lunch menu #9

Microwave Scrambled Egg (page 70)
on 1 slice whole wheat toast
with sliced tomatoes and lettuce

1 medium apple OR fruit of your choice (page 227)

3 graham wafers with 2 tbsp (25 mL) light cheese spread

1/2 cup (125 mL) low-fat milk

lunch menu #10

1 serving (1/4) **Luncheon Macaroni and Cheddar Cheese** (page 71)

1 serving (1/4) **Cabbage Waldorf Salad** (page 72)

herbal tea

lunch menu #11

1 cup (250 mL) **Curried Vegetable and Split Pea Soup** (page 73)

4 melba toasts with 2 tbsp (25 mL) light cream cheese

2/3 cup (150 mL) diced cantaloupe OR fruit of your choice (page 227)

1/2 cup (125 mL) low-fat milk

lunch menu #12

Tomato Beef Bouillon
*1/4 cup (50 mL) tomato juice, 1/2 cup (125 mL) beef bouillon
and 1/4 cup (50 mL) water, heated*

1 serving (1/4) **Egg Dill Sandwich Filling** (page 74)
on 2 slices rye bread (60 g)

1 serving (1/4) **Microwave Applesauce** (page 75)

1/2 cup (125 mL) low-fat milk

lunch menu #13

1 serving (1/2) **Fruit Plate with Ricotta Cheese** (page 76)

1/2 toasted bagel (45 g)
and 1/2 tsp (2 mL) soft margarine OR butter

tea or coffee with milk

lunch menu #14

1 serving (1/2) **Spicy Beans on Toast** (page 77)

sliced tomato and cucumber

2 small purple plums OR fruit of your choice (page 227)
1 wedge (25 g) light Cheddar cheese

1/2 cup (125 mL) low-fat milk

lunch menu #15

1 serving (1/2) **Chicken Caesar Salad Plate** (page 78)
with **Zesty Dressing** (page 79)

2 bread sticks (20 g)

1 wedge watermelon OR fruit of your choice (page 227)
1 chocolate-coated digestive cookie

diet soft drink

lunch menu #16

1 cup (250 mL) **Red Lentil and Barley Soup** (page 80)
with 2 tbsp (25 mL) low-fat plain yogurt

4 **Pita Cheese Crisps** (page 181)
1 wedge (25 g) light Cheddar cheese

1 medium raw apple or poached in 2 tbsp (25 mL) water with
dash cinnamon

tea or coffee with milk

lunch menu #17

1 serving (1/6) **Summertime Open-Faced Vegetable Sandwich** (page 81)

1/2 cup (125 mL) green or red grapes OR fruit of your choice (page 227)

Homemade Chocolate Milk
*blend 3/4 cup (175 mL) low-fat milk with 1 1/2 tsp (7 mL) cocoa,
sweetener and dash vanilla*

lunch menu #18

1 cup (250 mL) **Boston Clam Chowder** (page 82)

6 whole wheat crackers

1 kiwi fruit OR fruit of your choice (page 227)

lunch menu #19

1 serving (1/4) **Chicken Sandwich Filling** (page 83)
in 1 whole wheat pita (60 g), halved

1 large peach OR fruit of your choice (page 227)

1/2 cup (125 mL) low-fat milk

lunch menu #20

1 serving (1/2) **Creamed Salmon on Toast** (page 84)

1 small banana OR fruit of your choice (page 227)

1/2 cup (125 mL) low-fat milk

lunch menu #21

1 cup (250 mL) **Soup 'n Sandwich in a Bowl** (page 85)

1 large pear OR fruit of your choice (page 227)
2 whole meal digestive cookies

1/2 cup (125 mL) low-fat milk

lunch menu #22

1 serving (1/3) **Salmon Pecan Sandwich Filling** (page 86)
on 1 medium (90 g) bagel, sliced

sliced tomatoes and cucumbers

1 cup (250 mL) tomato juice

lunch menu #23

1 1/4 cups (300 mL) **Baked Bean Soup** (page 87)

1 slice whole wheat bread with 1 tsp (5 mL) soft margarine OR butter

1 orange, sliced
with 1/2 cup (125 mL) low-fat plain yogurt and dash cinnamon

lunch menu #24

1 cup (250 mL) **Gingered Carrot Soup** (page 88)

1 English muffin, halved; top with 1/3 cup (75 mL)
shredded light mozzarella cheese; broil until cheese melts

sliced cucumber

1 medium pear OR fruit of your choice (page 227)

tea or coffee with milk

lunch menu #25

1 serving (1/2) **Grilled Ham 'n Cheese French Toast Sandwich** (page 89)

2 slices fresh pineapple OR fruit of your choice (page 227)

1/2 cup (125 mL) low-fat milk

lunch menu #26

1 cup (250 mL) **Turkey Minestrone Soup** (page 90)

1 slice rye bread (30 g)
spread with 2 tbsp (25 mL) light cream cheese

2 medium plums OR fruit of your choice (page 227)

1/2 cup (125 mL) low-fat milk

lunch menu #27

1 serving (1/2) **Greek Salad in a Pita** (page 92)

1/2 orange and 1/4 cup (50 mL) seedless grapes

1/2 cup (125 mL) low-fat milk

lunch menu #28

1 cup (250 mL) **Hearty Vegetable Barley Soup** (page 93)

1 wedge (30 g) light Cheddar cheese
and 6 whole wheat soda crackers

1 mandarin orange OR fruit of your choice (page 227)
1 whole meal digestive cookie

1/2 cup (125 mL) low-fat milk

lunch menu #29

Broccoli and Rice Crustless Quiche (page 94)

1/2 tomato, sliced

1 medium pear OR fruit of your choice (page 227)
2 graham wafers

tea or coffee with milk

lunch menu #30

1 serving (1/2) **Cheesy Eggs with Asparagus on Toast** (page 95)

1 kiwi fruit and 1 orange, sliced

1/2 cup (125 mL) low-fat milk

lunch recipes index

lunch recipes

lunch menu #8

Tuna Sandwich Filling

Horseradish and parsley take common tuna filling to a new and enhanced taste level.

1	can (6 1/2 oz/184 g) water-packed chunk white tuna, drained	1
2 tbsp	low-fat (1%) plain yogurt	25 mL
2 tbsp	light mayonnaise	25 mL
1 tbsp	prepared horseradish	15 mL
2 tsp	chopped parsley	10 mL
Pinch	freshly ground pepper	Pinch

1 In bowl, flake tuna. Combine with yogurt, mayonnaise, horseradish, parsley and pepper. Cover and refrigerate for up to one day.

Makes 4 servings, 1 cup (250 mL).

lunch menu #8

Blender Yogurt Fruit Shake

This tasty fruit shake provides a beverage at lunch.

1	small banana	1
1 cup	fresh or frozen blueberries	250 mL
1 cup	low-fat (1%) plain yogurt	250 mL

1 In a blender container or food processor, blend banana, blueberries and yogurt until smooth.

Makes 2 servings, 2 cups (500 mL).

PREPARATION TIME:
10 minutes

CHILL:
up to one day

Each serving:
1/4 cup (50 mL) filling

1 1/2 PROTEIN CHOICES
1 EXTRA

2 g carbohydrate (0 g fibre)
10 g protein
3 g total fat (0 g saturated fat)
205 mg sodium
76 calories

KITCHEN TIP

Add extra crunch to sandwiches with alfalfa sprouts or pepper cress. Wash well before using.

Each serving:
1 cup (250 mL)

2 FRUITS & VEGETABLES CHOICES
1 1/2 MILK 1% CHOICES

30 g carbohydrate (3 g fibre)
7 g protein
3 g total fat (2 g saturated fat)
92 mg sodium
162 calories

PREPARATION TIME:
under 5 minutes

COOKING TIME:
about 50 seconds

Each serving:
1 egg

1 PROTEIN CHOICE
1 FATS & OILS CHOICE

1 g carbohydrate (0 g fibre)
6 g protein
7 g fat (2 g saturated fat)
89 mg sodium
92 calories

KITCHEN TIP

For additional servings, increase cooking time according to how many eggs are being prepared. See below.

2 eggs	2 tbsp (25 mL) water OR milk
	1 tsp (5 mL) soft margarine OR butter
	Cook for about 1 1/2 to 1 3/4 minutes
4 eggs	1/4 cup (50 mL) water OR milk
	2 tsp (10 mL) soft margarine OR butter
	Cook for 2 1/2 to 3 minutes
6 eggs	1/3 cup (75 mL) water OR milk
	1 tbsp (15 mL) soft margarine OR butter
	Cook for 3 to 3 1/2 minutes

lunch menu #9
Microwave Scrambled Egg

Eggs cooked in the microwave oven are a fast food at lunch or breakfast.

1/2 tsp	soft margarine OR butter	2 mL
1	egg	1
1 tbsp	water OR milk	15 mL

1 Melt margarine on High (100%) in large microwave-safe bowl. Stir in egg and water. Cover with plastic wrap. Microwave on Medium-High (70%) for about 50 seconds. Stir twice during cooking. Let stand for about 30 seconds before serving.

Makes 1 serving.

Variation: Seasoned Scrambled Egg

Vary flavours by adding seasonings such as dried basil or oregano; pinch dry mustard or ground nutmeg; celery or caraway seeds.

lunch menu #10

Luncheon Macaroni and Cheddar Cheese

Good old "mac 'n cheese" provides lots of comfort and flavour. This version reduces calories from fat.

1 tsp	soft margarine OR butter	5 mL
2 tbsp	finely chopped onion	25 mL
1	small clove garlic, minced	1
2 tbsp	all purpose flour	25 mL
2 cups	low-fat milk	500 mL
1/2 tsp	prepared OR dry mustard	2 mL
1/4 tsp	salt	1 mL
Dash	hot pepper sauce OR paprika	Dash
1 1/2 cups	shredded light Cheddar cheese	375 mL
1 1/4 cups	elbow macaroni	300 mL

1 In medium saucepan, melt margarine over low heat. Cook onion and garlic in margarine for 5 minutes; do not brown.

2 Whisk together flour, milk, mustard, salt and hot pepper sauce; gradually stir into onion. Cook over medium heat until mixture is smooth and thickened, stirring constantly. Add cheese; stir until melted.

3 In large amount of boiling water, cook macaroni according to package directions until al dente (tender but firm). Drain macaroni; add cheese sauce, toss well to combine. (See Tip.)

Makes 4 servings, 4 cups (1 L).

PREPARATION TIME:
10 minutes

COOKING TIME:
15 minutes

Each serving:
1 cup (250 mL)

2 STARCH CHOICES
1 MILK 2% CHOICE
2 PROTEIN CHOICES
1 FATS & OILS CHOICE

40 g carbohydrate (1 g fibre)
22 g protein
12 g total fat (7 g saturated fat)
533 mg sodium
361 calories

KITCHEN TIP

For any remaining macaroni and cheese, freeze in 1 cup (250 mL) amounts.

PREPARATION TIME:
15 minutes

CHILL:
30 minutes or longer

Each serving:
1 1/4 cups (300 mL)

2 FRUITS & VEGETABLES CHOICES
1 FATS & OILS CHOICE

19 g carbohydrate (3 g fibre)
2 g protein
5 g total fat (0 g saturated fat)
97 mg sodium
118 calories

Cabbage Waldorf Salad

This dressed-up cabbage salad is a good complement to chili for dinner or macaroni and cheese for lunch.

2 cups	coarsely shredded cabbage	500 mL
1/2 cup	sliced celery	125 mL
2 tbsp	each: finely chopped raisins and walnuts	25 mL
1/4 cup	low-fat (1%) plain yogurt	50 mL
2 tbsp	light mayonnaise	25 mL
1/2 tsp	lemon juice	2 mL
	Salt and pepper to taste	
2	medium apples, cored and chopped	2

1 In medium bowl, combine cabbage, celery, raisins and walnuts.

2 In a small bowl, whisk together yogurt, mayonnaise and lemon juice; stir into cabbage mixture. Season to taste with salt and pepper.

3 Cover and refrigerate for at least 30 minutes so flavours develop.

4 Stir in apple at serving time.

Makes 4 servings, 5 cups (1.25 L).

lunch menu #11

Curried Vegetable and Split Pea Soup

This wonderful wintertime soup tantalizes the taste buds with its subtle aromas and flavours. Since the recipe produces a large quantity of soup, freeze any leftover portion.

1 tbsp	canola oil	15 mL
1 cup	chopped onion (1 medium)	250 mL
2	cloves garlic, minced	2
2 tbsp	minced gingerroot OR 1 tsp (5 mL) ground ginger	25 mL
2	cinnamon sticks	2
2	bay leaves	2
1 tbsp	curry powder	15 mL
9 cups	chicken broth (see Tip)	2.25 L
2 cups	dry yellow split peas	500 mL
2 cups	chopped celery	500 mL
2 cups	finely chopped cauliflower	500 mL
1 1/2 cups	chopped carrot (3 medium)	375 mL
2 tbsp	tomato paste (see Tip)	25 mL
	Salt and pepper to taste	

1 In large, heavy saucepan, heat oil over medium heat. Add onion, garlic, gingerroot, cinnamon sticks and bay leaves. Cover and cook for 5 minutes or until vegetables are tender. Stir in curry powder and cook for 2 minutes.

2 Add chicken broth and split peas. Cover and simmer for 45 minutes or until peas are almost tender.

3 Add celery, cauliflower, carrot and tomato paste. Cover and simmer for 20 minutes or until peas and vegetables are tender. Season to taste with salt and pepper. Remove cinnamon sticks and bay leaves and discard.

Makes 12 servings, 12 cups (3 L).

PREPARATION TIME:
20 minutes

COOKING TIME:
1 hour and 10 minutes

Each serving:
1 cup (250 mL)

1 STARCH CHOICE
1/2 FRUITS & VEGETABLES CHOICE
1 1/2 PROTEIN CHOICES

26 g carbohydrate (6 g fibre)
13 g protein
3 g total fat (1 g saturated fat)
610 mg sodium
174 calories

KITCHEN TIPS

For chicken broth, use canned chicken broth OR prepare with chicken bouillon cubes OR **Homemade Chicken Broth** (page 91).

Tomato paste is often needed in small amounts, so freeze remaining from this recipe in ice cube trays in 1 or 2 tbsp (15 or 25 mL) amounts to use in other recipes.

PREPARATION TIME:
20 minutes

CHILL:
up to 1 day

Each serving:
1/3 cup (75 mL) filling

1 PROTEIN CHOICE
1 FATS & OILS CHOICE
1 EXTRA

2 g carbohydrate (0 g fibre)
7 g protein
7 g total fat (2 g saturated fat)
261 mg sodium
100 calories

KITCHEN TIP

Raw cucumber provides moisture and flavour to this filling with less mayonnaise and therefore fewer calories from fat.

lunch menu #12
Egg Dill Sandwich Filling

Prepared the night before, this sandwich filling will make short work of lunch preparation the next day.

4	hard cooked eggs, chopped	4
1/4 cup	finely chopped cucumber (see Tip)	50 mL
2 tbsp	light mayonnaise	25 mL
1/4 tsp	dried dill weed	1 mL
1/4 tsp	salt	1 mL
Pinch	freshly ground pepper	Pinch

1 In bowl, combine chopped eggs, cucumber, mayonnaise, dill weed, salt and pepper. Cover and refrigerate for up to one day.

Makes 4 servings, 1 1/3 cups (325 mL).

lunch menu #12

dinner menu #8

Microwave Applesauce

Warm applesauce, one of life's greatest comfort foods! Using the microwave oven gives us short cooking time and minimal cleanup.

3 1/2 cups	peeled, cored and sliced cooking apples (about 3 large Spy, Spartan or McIntosh)	875 mL
3/4 cup	water	175 mL
1/4 tsp	ground cinnamon	1 mL

1 In 6 cup (1.5 L) microwave-safe dish, combine apple slices and water. Cover and cook on High (100%) for 8 minutes or until apples are tender; stir once. Stir in cinnamon. Serve warm or at room temperature.

Makes 4 servings, 2 cups (500 mL).

PREPARATION TIME:
10 minutes

COOKING TIME:
8 minutes

Each serving:
1/2 cup (125 mL)

1 FRUITS & VEGETABLES CHOICE

14 g carbohydrate (2 g fibre)
0 g protein
0 g total fat
2 mg sodium
53 calories

PREPARATION TIME:
20 minutes

Each serving:
1/2 of recipe

2 FRUITS & VEGETABLES CHOICES
1/2 SUGARS CHOICE
1 MILK 2% CHOICE
1 1/2 PROTEIN CHOICES
1 FATS & OILS CHOICE

34 g carbohydrate (3 g fibre)
16 g protein
11 g total fat (6 g saturated fat)
165 mg sodium
282 calories

Fruit Plate with Ricotta Cheese

A variety of colourful fruits with ricotta cheese are a great choice when a friend comes for lunch

1 cup	light ricotta cheese	250 mL
2 tsp	finely grated orange rind	10 mL
2 tsp	granulated sugar	10 mL
1/8 tsp	each: ground ginger and nutmeg	0.5 mL
10	strawberries, sliced	10
2/3 cup	cantaloupe balls	150 mL
1/2 cup	halved green grapes	125 mL
1/4 cup	orange juice	50 mL
	Shredded lettuce	

1 In small bowl, stir together ricotta cheese, orange rind, sugar, ginger and nutmeg.

2 In second bowl, combine strawberries, cantaloupe, grapes and orange juice.

3 Arrange a bed of shredded lettuce on each of two serving plates. Top each with half of fruit mixture and half of the ricotta cheese. Serve at once.

Makes 2 servings.

lunch menu #14

Spicy Beans on Toast

Enhance a can of ordinary beans with spices and the fresh flavours of onion and parsley. Beans are a satisfying and slowly digested form of carbohydrate.

1 can	(14 oz/398 mL) vegetarian beans in tomato sauce	1
2	green onions, chopped	2
1/4 cup	chopped fresh parsley	50 mL
Pinch	each: garlic powder and chili powder	Pinch
Dash	Worcestershire sauce	Dash
2	slices whole wheat bread	2

1 In small saucepan, heat on medium-low beans, onions, parsley, garlic, chili powder and Worcestershire sauce until hot enough to serve.

2 Toast bread. Serve half of bean mixture over each toast slice.

Makes 2 servings.

PREPARATION TIME:
10 minutes

COOKING TIME:
about 5 minutes

Each serving:
1/2 of recipe over 1 slice toast

2 STARCH CHOICES
1 SUGARS CHOICE
1 1/2 PROTEIN CHOICES

59 g carbohydrate (17 g fibre)
14 g protein
2 g total fat (0 g saturated fat)
820 mg sodium
208 calories

PREPARATION TIME:
20 minutes

Each serving:
1/2 of recipe

**1 STARCH CHOICE
2 1/2 PROTEIN CHOICES**

17 g carbohydrate (2 g fibre)
20 g protein
7 g total fat (2 g saturated fat)
271 mg sodium
212 calories

lunch menu #15
Chicken Caesar Salad Plate

This simple version of the classic salad adds a touch of elegance to any lunch table.

1/2	cooked chicken breast (90 g), diced	1/2
4 cups	torn romaine lettuce	1 L
1 tbsp	grated Parmesan cheese	15 mL
2 tbsp	**Zesty Dressing** (page 79)	25 mL
1 cup	bread croutons	250 mL

1 In small bowl, combine chicken, lettuce and cheese. Drizzle with dressing; toss well.

2 Divide mixture onto two chilled salad plates. Top each with 1/2 cup (125 mL) bread croutons.

Makes 2 servings.

lunch menu #15

Zesty Dressing

Just as zesty as its name implies, this dressing adds zing to any salad.

2	flat anchovy fillets, optional	2
1	small clove garlic	1
1	egg white	1
2 tbsp	freshly grated Parmesan cheese	25 mL
1 1/2 tbsp	balsamic vinegar	22 mL
1 tbsp	fresh lime juice	15 mL
1/3 cup	chicken broth (see Tip)	75 mL
3 tbsp	olive oil	45 mL
1/8 tsp	freshly ground pepper	0.5 mL

1 Pat anchovies dry between paper towels. In food processor, process anchovies and garlic until finely chopped. Add egg white; process for 10 seconds. Add cheese, vinegar and lime juice; process until blended.

2 With machine running, slowly add chicken broth and oil until blended. Season with pepper.

3 Transfer dressing to a tightly closed container. Dressing can be refrigerated for up to one week; shake before using.

Makes 3/4 cup (175 mL).

PREPARATION TIME:
10 minutes

CHILL:
up to one week

Each serving:
1 tbsp (15 mL)

1/2 FATS & OILS CHOICE

0 g carbohydrate
1 g protein
3 g total fat (1 g saturated fat)
49 mg sodium
35 calories

KITCHEN TIP

Use canned chicken broth, OR reconstituted chicken bouillon cubes OR, of course, **Homemade Chicken Broth** (page 91) from backs and wings.

PREPARATION TIME:
20 minutes

COOKING TIME:
about 40 minutes

Each serving:
1 cup (250 mL)

1 STARCH CHOICE
1/2 FRUITS & VEGETABLES
CHOICE
1 PROTEIN CHOICE
1 EXTRA

29 g carbohydrate (7 g fibre)
8 g protein
3 g total fat (0 g saturated fat)
217 mg sodium
162 calories

KITCHEN TIP

Soups made with lentils and barley thicken when stored. You may need to add extra water or broth when reheating.

lunch menu #16

Red Lentil and Barley Soup

Lentils are a legume that, besides tasting great, are a powerhouse of fibre, vitamin A and iron. They are a complete protein when eaten with a grain like the barley in this soup. Red lentils cook faster than any other dried legume and do not require soaking (see Tip).

1 tbsp	olive oil	15 mL
1	large leek, thinly sliced (white part only)	1
1 cup	chopped onion (1 large)	250 mL
3	cloves garlic, minced	3
6 cups	beef OR vegetable broth	1.5 L
1 3/4 cups	cubed carrots (4 medium)	425 mL
1 cup	sliced celery (2 stalks with leaves)	250 mL
3/4 cup	red lentils, washed	175 mL
3/4 cup	barley, washed	175 mL
1/2 cup	tomato sauce	125 mL
2	bay leaves	2
1 tsp	each: dried rosemary and oregano	5 mL
1/2 tsp	salt	2 mL
1/4 tsp	freshly ground pepper	1 mL
	Chopped fresh parsley	

1 In large soup pot, heat oil on medium-low heat; cook leek, onion and garlic, covered, for 10 minutes. Add broth, carrots, celery, lentils, barley, tomato sauce, bay leaves, rosemary, oregano, salt and pepper.

2 Cover and bring to a boil; reduce heat and simmer for 40 minutes or until barley is tender, stirring occasionally. Discard bay leaves. Serve sprinkled with parsley.

Makes 9 servings, 9 cups (2.25 L).

lunch menu #17

Summertime Open-Faced Vegetable Sandwich

This recipe draws rave reviews every time we serve it. We call it "summertime" since this is when we first tried it, but it can be enjoyed in the winter too. And, one serving is a good source of vitamin C.

1	round Italian-style gourmet flatbread (about 14 oz /400 g)	1
1/2 cup	cream cheese with onion dip (see Tip)	125 mL
1 cup	small broccoli florets	250 mL
1	small tomato, finely diced	1
2 tbsp	chopped red onion	25 mL
3/4 cup	thinly sliced mushrooms	175 mL
1/2 cup	diced red, yellow or green sweet pepper	125 mL
1 1/2 cups	shredded light Cheddar cheese (100 g)	375 mL
2 tbsp	sliced black olives	25 mL

1 Place flatbread on large serving dish. Spread evenly with dip.

2 Blanch broccoli in boiling water for 2 minutes; remove and chill under cold running water to stop cooking; drain. Randomly scatter broccoli, tomato, onion, mushrooms, sweet pepper, cheese and olives over dip. Cover and refrigerate for 1 hour or up to 8 hours. To serve, cut into 6 wedges.

Makes 6 servings.

PREPARATION TIME:
15 minutes

CHILL:
1 hour or longer

Each serving:
1/6 of recipe

2 STARCH CHOICES
1/2 FRUITS & VEGETABLES CHOICE
1 1/2 PROTEIN CHOICES
1 FATS & OILS CHOICE

37 g carbohydrate (3 g fibre)
13 g protein
10 g total fat (4 g saturated fat)
640 mg sodium
289 calories

KITCHEN TIP

Onion dip is usually found in 227 g packages. This recipe uses only 1/2 cup (125 mL), about 1/2 of the package.

PREPARATION TIME:
10 minutes

COOKING TIME:
about 15 minutes

Each serving:
1 cup (250 mL)

1 STARCH CHOICE
1 1/2 MILK 2% CHOICES
2 PROTEIN CHOICES
1 EXTRA

27 g carbohydrate (2 g fibre)
23 g protein
4 g total fat (2 g saturated fat)
388 mg sodium
241 calories

lunch menu #18
Boston Clam Chowder

Of all chowders, clam is probably the best known. Low-fat evaporated milk gives this version its rich creamy taste. One serving is an excellent source of iron, riboflavin, vitamins B12 and D.

2	slices lean side bacon	2
1/2 cup	minced celery	125 mL
1/4 cup	finely chopped onion	50 mL
2	cans (5 oz/142 g) baby clams	2
1 1/4 cups	cubed potatoes, (2 medium)	300 mL
1/4 tsp	each: salt, pepper, dried thyme leaves	1 mL
1	can (385 mL) low-fat evaporated milk	1

1 In saucepan, cook bacon until crisp; drain on paper towel and crumble. Set aside. Pour off bacon fat and discard. Add celery and onion; cook for 5 minutes or until tender.

2 Drain clams; reserve liquid, adding water to make 1 cup (250 mL), if needed. Add clam liquid, potato, salt, pepper and thyme. Cover and cook over medium heat for 10 minutes or until potato is tender. Add clams, bacon and milk. Heat over low heat to serving temperature.

Makes 5 servings, 5 cups (1.25 L).

lunch menu #19

Chicken Sandwich Filling

Sandwiches are still one of the fastest meals to prepare and one of the most portable. Chicken filling is an all-time favourite and a great way to use cooked chicken (or turkey).

1 1/2 cups	diced cooked chicken	375 mL
1/2 cup	diced celery (1 stalk)	125 mL
1/4 cup	thinly sliced green onions (2)	50 mL
1/4 cup	diced sweet orange OR green pepper	50 mL
3 tbsp	toasted slivered almonds	45 mL
1/4 cup	low-fat (1%) plain yogurt	50 mL
2 tbsp	light mayonnaise	25 mL
1 tbsp	chopped fresh tarragon OR 1 tsp (5 mL) dried (see Tip)	15 mL
Pinch	each: salt and pepper	Pinch

1 In bowl, combine chicken, celery, onions, orange pepper and almonds.

2 Whisk together yogurt, mayonnaise, tarragon, salt and pepper. Stir into chicken mixture. Cover and refrigerate for up to two days.

Makes 4 servings, 2 cups (500 mL).

PREPARATION TIME:
15 minutes

CHILL:
up to 2 days

Each serving:
1/2 cup (125 mL)

2 PROTEIN CHOICES
1 FATS & OILS CHOICE
1 EXTRA

4 g carbohydrate (1 g fibre)
13 g protein
10 g total fat (2 g saturated fat)
157 mg sodium
153 calories

KITCHEN TIP

Try curry powder as an interesting replacement for tarragon.

PREPARATION TIME:
10 minutes

COOKING TIME:
about 5 minutes

Each serving:
1/2 recipe

2 STARCH CHOICES
1/2 FRUITS & VEGETABLES
CHOICE
2 PROTEIN CHOICES
1 FATS & OILS CHOICE

40 g carbohydrate (6 g fibre)
18 g protein
11 g total fat (2 g saturated fat)
1573 mg sodium
327 calories

lunch menu #20
Creamed Salmon on Toast

Your mother probably served you this delightful comforting dish when she was pressed for time to make lunch.

1	can (10 oz/284 mL) half-fat cream of mushroom condensed soup	1
1/2 cup	canned salmon, undrained	125 mL
1/2 cup	frozen peas	125 mL
4	slices whole wheat bread	4

1 In small saucepan or microwave-safe bowl, combine soup, salmon and peas. Heat on medium, stirring frequently until peas are cooked and mixture is hot. Add water if needed to thin to serving consistency.

2 Toast bread. Serve half salmon over 2 slices of toast.

Makes 2 servings.

lunch menu #21

Soup 'n Sandwich in a Bowl

This is a novel way to eat your soup and sandwich at the same time.

1	can (28 oz/798 mL) diced tomatoes, undrained	1
1	can (10 oz/284 mL) condensed tomato soup	1
2/3 cup	water	150 mL
1 tsp	dried basil	5 mL
1/4 tsp	garlic powder	1 mL
1/4 tsp	freshly ground pepper	1 mL
5	slices whole wheat bread	5
1/2 cup	shredded light Cheddar cheese	125 mL
1	green onion, chopped	1

1 In 8 cup (2 L) microwave-safe casserole, combine tomatoes with juice, tomato soup, water, basil, garlic powder and pepper. Cover and microwave on High (100%) for 7 minutes or until soup is hot.

2 Toast bread; cut each slice into cubes. Spoon 1 cup (250 mL) soup into each of 5 bowls.

3 Top each bowl with cubes from 1 slice of toast. Sprinkle each with about 2 tbsp (25 mL) cheese and some chopped green onion. Microwave for a few seconds until cheese melts.

Makes 5 servings, 5 cups (1.25 L).

PREPARATION TIME:
15 minutes

COOKING TIME:
7 minutes

Each serving:
1 cup (250 mL)

1 STARCH CHOICE
1/2 FRUITS & VEGETABLES CHOICE
1/2 SUGARS CHOICE
1 PROTEIN CHOICE

30 g carbohydrate (5 g fibre)
9 g protein
4 g total fat (2 g saturated fat)
920 mg sodium
179 calories

PREPARATION TIME:
10 minutes

CHILL:
up to two days

Each serving:
1/2 cup (125 mL)

1 1/2 PROTEIN CHOICES
1 1/2 FATS & OILS CHOICES
1 EXTRA

2 g carbohydrate (0 g fibre)
12 g protein
12 g total fat (2 g saturated fat)
352 mg sodium
163 calories

KITCHEN TIPS

For a calcium boost, we've recommended that you mash the bones with the salmon. This provides as much extra calcium as a small glass of milk.

To toast nuts, place pecans on a microwave-safe dish. Microwave on High (100%) for about 1 minute. Watch carefully as they will brown very quickly.

lunch menu #22

Salmon Pecan Sandwich Filling

The toasted nutty flavour and crunch of pecans make the difference in our version of this ever-favourite sandwich filling. Omega-3 fatty acids found in salmon make this filling "heart-healthy."

1	can (7.5 oz/213 g) salmon, undrained (see Tip)	1
2 tbsp	light mayonnaise	25 mL
1 tsp	horseradish	5 mL
2	green onions, finely chopped	2
1 tbsp	toasted chopped pecans (see Tip)	15 mL
	Chopped parsley, optional	

1 In bowl, flake salmon, remove skin and discard; mash bones with salmon (see Tip). Stir in mayonnaise, horseradish, onions, pecans and parsley, if using. Cover and refrigerate for up to two days.

Makes 3 servings, 1 1/2 cups (375 mL).

lunch menu #23

Baked Bean Soup

When your time is limited, this vegetarian recipe provides a fast, simple and nutritious lunch.

1	can (19 oz/540 mL) diced tomatoes	1
1	can (14 oz/398 mL) vegetarian beans in tomato sauce	1
1 cup	water	250 mL
1/4 cup	chopped onion	50 mL
1/2 tsp	dried oregano	2 mL
1/4 tsp	dry mustard	1 mL
1/2 cup	shredded light mozzarella cheese	125 mL

1 In medium saucepan, combine tomatoes, beans, water, onion, oregano and mustard. Cover and cook on medium heat for 15 minutes or until hot and onion is tender.

2 Sprinkle each serving with 2 tbsp (25 mL) cheese.

Makes 4 servings, 5 cups (1.25 L).

PREPARATION TIME:
10 minutes

COOKING TIME:
15 minutes

Each serving:
1 1/4 cups (300 mL)

1/2 STARCH CHOICE
1/2 FRUITS & VEGETABLES CHOICE
1/2 SUGARS CHOICE
1 PROTEIN CHOICE

29 g carbohydrate (10 g fibre)
10 g protein
3 g total fat (2 g saturated fat)
722 mg sodium
171 calories

PREPARATION TIME:
20 minutes

COOKING TIME:
about 30 minutes

Each serving:
1 cup (250 mL)

1 FRUITS & VEGETABLES CHOICE
1/2 MILK 2% CHOICE
1/2 PROTEIN CHOICE
1 EXTRA

18 g carbohydrate (3 g fibre)
7 g protein
4 g total fat (1 g saturated fat)
583 mg sodium
129 calories

Variation: Cold Gingered Carrot Soup
Refrigerate extra soup to serve cold or freeze for later use.

KITCHEN TIPS

Peeling fresh gingerroot can be a chore. Use a blunt-edged teaspoon to scrape away peel with speedy and efficient results.

To keep carrots moist and vitamin-rich, chop off their green tops before refrigerating in plastic bags.

lunch menu #24
Gingered Carrot Soup

The spicy scent of ginger added to this heart-warming soup fills the air with exciting aromas any time of the year.

1 tbsp	soft margarine OR butter	15 mL
1 cup	finely chopped onion	250 mL
1	leek, white and light green part only, chopped	1
1	stalk celery, finely chopped	1
1 tbsp	finely chopped gingerroot (see Tip)	15 mL
1	clove garlic, minced	1
6	large carrots, peeled and chopped (3 1/4 cups/800 mL) (see Tip)	6
4 cups	chicken OR vegetable broth	1 L
1	can (160 mL) 2% evaporated milk	1
	Freshly ground pepper, to taste	
	Chopped fresh parsley	

1 In large saucepan, on medium heat, melt margarine. Add onion, leek and celery; sauté for 5 minutes. Add gingerroot and garlic; sauté for 1 minute. Add carrots and broth; bring to a boil, reduce heat, cover and simmer for 30 minutes or until vegetables are tender. Remove pan from heat and cool slightly.

2 Purée soup in batches in food processor or blender until very smooth. Return to saucepan, slowly bring to boil and add milk, stirring frequently to prevent sticking. Before serving, stir and check seasonings, then season to taste with pepper. Sprinkle each serving with chopped parsley.

Makes 6 servings, 6 cups (1.5 L).

lunch menu #25

Grilled Ham 'n Cheese French Toast Sandwich

This is an interesting combination of traditional French toast and a traditional grilled cheese sandwich. Using whole wheat bread makes it a high source of fibre.

4	slices whole wheat bread	4
1 tbsp	Dijon mustard	15 mL
1 tsp	light mayonnaise	5 mL
2	slices lean ham (60 g)	2
2	thin slices (40 g) light processed Cheddar cheese	2
1	egg OR 2 egg whites	1
2 tbsp	low-fat milk	25 mL
1/8 tsp	freshly ground pepper	0.5 mL

1 Place bread slices on cutting board. Combine mustard and mayonnaise; brush over two bread slices.

2 Arrange 1 slice meat and 1 slice cheese on 2 bread slices. Top with remaining 2 bread slices.
In shallow bowl or pie plate, whisk together egg, milk and pepper. Dip sandwiches in egg mixture; allow sandwiches to remain in mixture until all liquid is absorbed.

3 Heat medium non-stick skillet on medium-high. Lightly spray with non-stick cooking spray. Place each sandwich in skillet; cook for 5 minutes or until browned on both sides and cheese melts.

Makes 2 sandwiches.

PREPARATION TIME:
5 minutes

COOKING TIME:
about 5 minutes

Each serving:
1 sandwich

2 STARCH CHOICES
2 1/2 PROTEIN CHOICES
1/2 FATS & OILS CHOICE

33 g carbohydrate (5 g fibre)
22 g protein
11 g total fat (3 g saturated fat)
1120 mg sodium
310 calories

PREPARATION TIME:
15 minutes

COOKING TIME:
about 15 minutes

Each serving:
1 cup (250 mL)

1 STARCH CHOICE
1/2 FRUITS & VEGETABLES
CHOICE
2 PROTEIN CHOICES

25 g carbohydrate (3 g fibre)
16 g protein
4 g total fat (1 g saturated fat)
743 mg sodium
196 calories

KITCHEN TIP

Guidelines recommend using less salt and sodium as this may help prevent hypertension or high blood pressure (see page 7). Rinsing canned beans lowers the sodium content of a recipe. So does using a sodium-reduced broth, like **Homemade Chicken Broth** (page 91).

lunch menu #26
Turkey Minestrone Soup

Minestrone is a thick vegetable soup containing pasta and beans, adding slowly digested carbohydrate and fibre to this hearty soup.

1 tsp	canola oil	5 mL
1/2 cup	diced zucchini	125 mL
1/4 cup	chopped onion	50 mL
1	clove garlic, minced	1
2 cups	chicken broth (see Tip)	500 mL
2/3 cup	canned crushed tomatoes	150 mL
2/3 cup	drained rinsed pinto OR romano beans (see Tip)	150 mL
1/4 cup	elbow macaroni	50 mL
1/4 tsp	each: dried oregano and basil	1 mL
1/2 cup	diced cooked turkey OR chicken	125 mL
	Chopped fresh parsley, optional	

1 In saucepan, heat oil over medium heat. Add zucchini, onion and garlic. Cook for 5 minutes or until softened.

2 Stir in broth, tomatoes and beans. Bring to boil, add oregano, basil and macaroni; cover, reduce heat and cook gently for 12 minutes or until macaroni is tender. Add turkey; heat to serving temperature. Before serving, stir soup and check seasonings. It may need extra oregano or basil. Sprinkle each serving with parsley, if using.

3 Remember that on standing, pasta continues to soften and absorb liquid. If the soup is too thick after standing, add extra stock or water.

Makes 3 servings, about 3 cups (750 mL).

Homemade Chicken Broth

Any recipe calling for chicken broth will only be as good as the broth you use. Our **Homemade Chicken Broth** will give your recipes maximum flavour with much less sodium than commercial varieties.

TO PREPARE:

Store poultry bones in freezer until enough are accumulated to make a quantity of broth. The more bones, the better the flavour. Place the frozen bones, along with any fresh ones you may have on hand, in a large saucepan.

Add enough cold water to cover the bones by 1 inch (2.5 cm). Add 1 chopped onion, 2 stalks chopped celery and 2 sprigs fresh parsley and a bay leaf. Bring to boil, cover, reduce heat and simmer for 2 hours or longer. Strain, discard bones and chill liquid. When broth is cold, remove any congealed fat and discard. Measure and freeze in appropriate amounts to use as needed.

S O D I U M   T I P

How much sodium is in chicken broth? Read labels and compare.

homemade chicken broth	15 mg per cup (250 mL)
canned chicken broth (25% less sodium)	610 mg per cup (250 mL)
ready-to-use broth in cartons (25% less sodium)	638 mg per cup (250 mL)
ready-to-use broth in cartons (regular)	972 mg per cup (250 mL)
chicken bouillon sachet (makes 3/4 cup [175 mL]) (35% less salt)	527 mg

PREPARATION TIME:
15 minutes

Each serving:
1/2 of recipe

2 STARCH CHOICES
1 FRUITS & VEGETABLES CHOICE
1 1/2 PROTEIN CHOICES
1 1/2 FATS & OILS CHOICES

45 g carbohydrate (**8 g fibre**)
14 g protein
12 g total fat (4 g saturated fat)
743 mg sodium
327 calories

Greek Salad in a Pita

A pita pocket holds a Greek salad to make this sandwich a possibility.

2	sliced tomatoes	2
1 cup	diced cucumber	250 mL
6	Kalamata olives, sliced	6
1/2 cup	crumbled feta cheese	125 mL
2 tbsp	lemon juice	25 mL
2 tsp	olive oil	10 mL
	Shredded romaine lettuce	
4	whole wheat pita bread halves (60 g each)	4

1 In a medium bowl, combine tomatoes, cucumber, olives and cheese. Toss with lemon juice and oil.

2 Place shredded lettuce into each pita bread half. Evenly divide cucumber mixture over lettuce in each pita.

Makes 2 servings, 4 pita halves.

lunch menu #28

Hearty Vegetable Barley Soup

Barley, like oats, is an excellent source of soluble fibre as well as low glycemic index carbohydrate (see page 4). Pot barley is less refined and more nutritious than pearl barley.

1/2 cup	chopped onion	125 mL
1	can (10 oz/284 mL) condensed beef broth (see Tip)	1
1 cup	water	250 mL
1/4 cup	pot barley	50 mL
2/3 cup	cubed potato (1 medium)	150 mL
1/2 cup	chopped carrot	125 mL
1	stalk celery, diced	1
1/2 cup	cubed rutabaga	125 mL
1	bay leaf	1
1/2 tsp	dried thyme	2 mL
Pinch	each: salt and freshly ground pepper	Pinch
	Chopped fresh parsley, optional	

1 In medium saucepan, combine onion, broth, water and barley. Bring to a boil, reduce heat, cover and simmer for 45 minutes.

2 Add potato, carrot, celery, rutabaga, bay leaf, thyme, salt and pepper. Cook for 15 minutes or until vegetables are tender. Before serving, stir soup, taste and adjust seasoning. You may need to add extra thyme. Serve soup with chopped parsley, if using.

Makes 3 servings, 3 cups (750 mL).

PREPARATION TIME:
15 minutes

COOKING TIME:
about 1 hour

Each serving:
1 cup (250 mL)

1 STARCH CHOICE
1/2 FRUITS & VEGETABLES CHOICE
1/2 PROTEIN CHOICE
1 EXTRA

26 g carbohydrate (5 g fibre)
8 g protein
1 g total fat (0 g saturated fat)
525 mg sodium
136 calories

KITCHEN TIP

For a vegetarian version, substitute vegetable broth made with vegetable bouillon cubes.

PREPARATION TIME:
15 minutes

COOKING TIME:
about 30 minutes

Each serving:
1 recipe

1 STARCH CHOICE
1/2 FRUITS & VEGETABLES
CHOICE
1 MILK 1% CHOICE
2 PROTEIN CHOICES
1 FATS & OILS CHOICE

26 g carbohydrate (**3 g fibre**)
21 g protein
11 g total fat (6 g saturated fat)
416 mg sodium
290 calories

lunch menu #29

Broccoli and Rice Crustless Quiche

Eliminating the crust leaves us with all the flavour of a great quiche but without the high fat found in pastry. Using a lower-fat cheese reduces calories even further.

1	egg OR 2 egg whites	1
1 tsp	Dijon mustard	5 mL
1/4 tsp	dried basil	1 mL
1/8 tsp	each: salt and freshly ground pepper	0.5 mL
1 tbsp	each: finely chopped onion and sweet red pepper	15 mL
1/4 cup	shredded light Swiss cheese	50 mL
1/2 cup	low-fat milk	125 mL
1/2 cup	chopped broccoli	125 mL
1/2 cup	cooked brown OR white rice (see Tip)	125 mL

1 Lightly spray shallow 2 cup (500 mL) casserole with non-stick vegetable spray.

2 In small bowl, beat egg, mustard, basil, salt and pepper until well blended. Add onion, red pepper and cheese; mix well.

3 In microwave, heat milk on High (100%) for 30 seconds or until very warm, but not boiling. Stir hot milk into broccoli and rice. Slowly add egg mixture, stirring constantly.

4 Pour into prepared pan. Bake in 350°F (180°C) oven for 30 minutes or until knife inserted in centre comes out clean. Let stand for 5 minutes before serving.

Makes 1 serving.

lunch menu #30

Cheesy Eggs with Asparagus on Toast

This wonderful recipe is especially appropriate in spring when fresh, tender shoots of asparagus are readily available.

Cheese Sauce

2 tsp	cornstarch	10 mL
1/4 tsp	dry mustard	1 mL
1/8 tsp	each: salt and pepper	0.5 mL
3/4 cup	low-fat milk	175 mL
1/4 cup	shredded light Cheddar cheese	50 mL
1 tsp	soft margarine OR butter	5 mL
2	hard-cooked eggs	2
10	asparagus stalks	10
2	slices whole wheat toast	2
	Paprika	

1 In 1 cup (250 mL) glass measure, combine cornstarch, mustard, salt and pepper. Slowly whisk in milk. Microwave on High (100%) for 1 minute; stir well. Microwave on Medium-High (70%) for 2 minutes or until sauce begins to thicken. Stir cheese and margarine into sauce, stirring until melted.

2 Remove shells from eggs and slice. Steam asparagus.

3 Divide eggs and asparagus over each slice of toast. Spoon cheese sauce over eggs and asparagus; sprinkle with paprika.

Makes 2 servings and 3/4 cup (175 mL) sauce.

PREPARATION TIME:
10 minutes

COOKING TIME:
about 3 minutes

Each serving:
1/2 of recipe

1 STARCH CHOICE
1 MILK 1% CHOICE
1 1/2 PROTEIN CHOICES
1 FATS & OILS CHOICE
1 EXTRA

23 g carbohydrate (2 g fibre)
16 g protein
10 g total fat (3 g saturated fat)
465 mg sodium
242 calories

dinner

Dinner is a time to relax after the day's activities and wind down with a pleasant and satisfying meal. For most, it is the major meal of the day, and that's the way our menus treat it. Our recipes follow the healthiest and lowest-fat cooking methods: broiling, microwaving, steaming and stir-frying. Dinner is traditionally a meal of a meat (the protein), potatoes (the starch), some other vegetables and a dessert. When planning dinner, we tend to first question the protein portion of the meal—will it be poultry, fish, meat or a meat alternative? But remember that protein is only a small part of a healthy meal. We should question what vegetables and starches we will eat and then fit in an appropriate protein choice. Think of your dinner plate as half covered by vegetables, one-quarter covered by starch and one-quarter covered by protein.

How Much?

Some of the prepared foods in the menus and recipes need to be measured so you know you have the right amount on your plate. We suggest you have a set of graduated "dry" measuring cups—the ones in 1/4 cup, 1/3 cup, 1/2 cup and 1 cup (or 50 mL, 75 mL, 125 mL and 250 mL) sizes. These are also useful for measuring dry ingredients in recipes, so do double duty. Two or three pyrex "liquid" measuring cups in 1 cup, 2 cup and possibly 4 cup (or 250 mL, 500 mL and 1L) sizes come in handy as well. Having measures at hand speeds up serving meals.

Vegetables

Let's start with how we fill half the plate. What are vegetables and why are they so important?

Vegetables are the cornerstone of any healthy meal, especially if you have diabetes. They supply us with nearly all the vitamins, minerals and fibre essential to good health. Potatoes and corn, from a diabetes point of view, are not vegetables, but starches. But tomatoes, eggplant, squashes and peppers, considered fruits by botanists, are considered to be vegetables by the rest of us. Everything else we have always thought were vegetables probably are vegetables!

All living plants produce carbohydrate and store it in their roots or fruit in the form of starch or sugar. Vegetables that are the leaf, stem or flower of a plant or are very young contain only a small amount. In the diabetes world these are called "EXTRA VEGETABLES." Root vegetables, and other vegetables that must ripen, contain more carbohydrate because they have more time to store it. These vegetables are often sweet tasting like fruit, so in the diabetes world they are called "FRUITS AND VEGETABLES."

Vegetables are considered to be "nutrient dense," that is, they have a high amount of nutrients for the number of calories they supply. Considering the cost of most vegetables relative to meats, they are a magnificent nutrition bargain!

Facts about EXTRA VEGETABLES

Asparagus: Asparagus contains a good supply of vitamins and minerals. For microwave directions, see page 100. Or cook asparagus, covered and upright, in a small amount of boiling water for 3 to 5 minutes.

Broccoli: Some call it "green goodness" and certainly it boasts more nutrients than almost any other vegetable, especially calcium and beta-carotene (vitamin A). Peel stalks if they are tough, but be sure to include the tender leaves. Steam for 5 to 7 minutes.

Cabbage: Along with vitamin C, cabbage contains fibre. Steam quartered or sliced cabbage for about 10 minutes; shredded cabbage for 5 to 10 minutes.

Green Beans: Beans contain good amounts of beta-carotene and vitamin C. Since they are immature, they are low in carbohydrate. Trim stem ends only; cover and steam or boil for 3 to 5 minutes.

Leeks: They are prized for their subtle onion flavour and rich folate content. Steam cut-up leeks for 3 to 5 minutes, whole for 10 to 15 minutes.

Mushrooms: Mushrooms grow in the dark and so have little or no carbohydrate. Sauté mushrooms, uncovered, with a little broth or olive oil. Cook on medium-high for 3 to 5 minutes until all liquid is evaporated. Cooked fresh mushrooms have far more nutrients than canned.

Onions: Sliced, chopped, grated or diced, onions add flavour to a dish. They are cooked in many ways, based on the recipe being prepared. Since they are low in nutrients, the cooking method is not a concern.

Sweet and Hot Peppers: Like onions, peppers can be chopped, diced and sliced. They are very rich in beta-carotene and add flavour as well as colour to many dishes. Peppers are great sautéed, stir-fried or stuffed.

Snow Peas: Snow peas should be shiny and flat. The smallest ones are sweetest and most tender. Remove tips and strings from both ends of the pod, cover and steam for 1 to 2 minutes to retain vitamin C (see page 101 for microwave instructions).

Spinach and Swiss Chard: Select small leaves with good green colour and thin stems. Wash, but do not dry. Steam for about 5 minutes. Greens are rich in vitamin A, folic acid and iron, but little of the iron content is available to us due to the presence of oxalic acid.

Tomatoes: Wonderful served raw with basil, they can also be baked, broiled or sautéed. See **Baked Eggs with Tomato** (page 152).

Zucchini: High in water content, zucchini is very low in calories. Cut into 1/4 inch (6 mm) slices and steam or sauté for 3 to 5 minutes (see **Vegetable Kebabs**, page 147).

Facts about FRUITS AND VEGETABLES

Carrots: They are one of the best sources of beta-carotene and one of the least expensive. **Gingered Carrot Soup** (page 88) is a great use for this humble vegetable.

Green Peas: Fresh peas have a very short season and most are sold frozen. The smaller the size, the better the flavour and the more tender. Steam peas for 5 to 10 minutes. They are a good source of protein and vitamin C. Frozen green peas retain their colour, flavour and nutrients better than canned and are low in sodium.

Parsnips: Considered a cold weather root vegetable and a cousin to the carrot, they are easy to prepare and are a good source of vitamin C. Steaming is the best way to cook them. But parsnips are also delicious roasted alone or with other vegetables, as in **Oven-Roasted Winter Vegetables** (page 120).

Rutabagas: Some people still think of rutabagas as turnips, but they are two very different vegetables. Rutabagas are larger with a yellow flesh and turnips are smaller and white-fleshed. Cut up, they are then boiled for 7 to 10 minutes. Rutabagas are the best source of vitamin C of all the root vegetables and contain beta-carotene.

Winter Squash: An excellent source of beta-carotene, these squash are hard-shelled with long keeping qualities. A very versatile vegetable, squash can be baked, boiled, microwaved, steamed, or cooked in a stovetop stew with chicken, as in **Herbed Chicken and Vegetables** (page 161).

What Is the Best Way to Cook Vegetables?

We have developed the "rule of least" for cooking vegetables—the least peeling, least amount of cooking water, least time to cook, and least waiting time after cooking. Vegetable skins contain nutrients and fibre, so peeling should be done only when absolutely necessary. Completely submerging vegetables in water, boiling, then draining removes most (if not all) of the water-soluble vitamins such as vitamin C, thiamin, niacin, B6, B12 and folacin. The longer vegetables are boiled, the more vitamin C is destroyed.

The microwave is perfect for vegetable cookery since vegetables retain more nutrients and microwaving is fast. Stir-frying is also excellent for the same reasons. Steaming uses a minimum of water and is almost as good as the other two methods. Maybe most importantly, vegetables are at their flavour peak when cooked tender-crisp. When vegetables are not served immediately after cooking, they lose flavour as well as nutrients.

Microwave cooking directions

Use only a sprinkle of water. Cover vegetables while microwaving to reduce cooking time and nutrient loss. Cook most vegetables quickly at High (100%). Don't overcook; instead use the recommended standing time to finish the cooking.

Here are directions for cooking single-serving amounts of some commonly used vegetables. All should stand for 3 to 5 minutes after cooking and before serving. (Microwave cooking continues for a short period after the microwave shuts off and food is removed from the oven.)

Asparagus: Trim 6 spears, place in microwave dish with tips facing inward. Sprinkle with water, cover and cook on High (100%) 1 1/2 to 2 minutes.

Beans: Trim beans, place in microwave dish. Sprinkle with water, cover and cook on High about 5 minutes.

Broccoli: Arrange trimmed stalks facing outward in microwave dish. Sprinkle with water, cover and cook on High 3 to 4 minutes.

Carrots: Remove thin peel from carrots and slice (young new carrots require no peeling). Place in microwave dish, sprinkle with water, cover and cook on Medium (50%) 5 minutes or until tender.

Rutabaga (*Turnip*): For mashed rutabaga, there's no need to peel or chop before cooking. With a knife, prick rutabaga in several places. Wrap in paper towel, place in microwave dish; cook on High (100%), turning halfway through. For 2.2 lb (1 kg) size, allow 14 to 17 minutes. Let stand 10 minutes before peeling.

Snow Peas: Trim by removing stems and strings along both sides of pods. Place in microwave dish, sprinkle with water, cover and cook on High (100%) 1 to 1 1/2 minutes.

Squash: Cut in half lengthwise and remove seeds; peel and chop into small cubes. Place in microwave dish, sprinkle with water, cover and cook on High (100%) 1 1/2 to 2 minutes or until tender.

Baked Potato: Wash 1 medium potato, pierce in several places with a fork. Place uncovered in microwave dish. Cook on High (100%) 4 to 6 minutes.

Are Some Vegetables Better for Me Than Others?

Many commonly used vegetables are a powerhouse of vitamins and minerals. The most nutritious vegetables are: broccoli, spinach, Brussels sprouts, lima beans, peas, asparagus, artichokes, cauliflower, sweet potatoes and carrots, rated on their content of vitamin A, thiamin, niacin, riboflavin, vitamin C, potassium, iron and calcium.

Facts about STARCH FOODS

Starchy carbohydrates (carbohydrate stored as starch in plants) are the single most important source of food energy in the world and are our bodies' principal source of energy. Since the carbohydrate we eat also has a major impact on blood glucose levels, this food group is very important for people with diabetes. It needs to be part of every meal, but in limited amounts. Our dinner menus and recipes use a variety of STARCH FOODS, with emphasis on slowly digested ones such as rice and pasta and potatoes, both white and sweet.

Potatoes: Potatoes are tubers, swollen underground stems that store surplus starch in order to feed the above ground plants. Few foods are as wholesome as a potato. Carbohydrates, vitamins (particularly C) and minerals—the potato has them all in ample amounts and some protein as well. Many consider potatoes fattening. Not so—the only fat is what you add in cooking or at the table. Properly prepared, we feel potatoes taste so good they really don't need much of anything.

The best way to prepare potatoes is to cook them in their skins. The skin is an excellent source of fibre, and many of the nutrients are just below the skin. So simply scrub unpeeled potatoes under cold water before cooking. If you must peel them, use a vegetable peeler to remove the thinnest possible layer of skin.

There are so many great ways to cook potatoes. Grilled on the barbecue, baked in the oven (see **Roasted Rosemary Potatoes**, page 159) or scalloped as in **Scalloped Sweet and White Potatoes** (page 154). Sweet potatoes, with their dense fluffy texture, are great cooked in the microwave, as are Yukon Gold potatoes.

Microwaving Tips

It is important to place potatoes on a paper towel to absorb moisture produced as the potato cooks. Prick in several places to allow steam to escape. Cook on High (100 %).

Number of Potatoes	Arrangement in Oven	Baking Time (Minutes)
1	centre	4–5
2	side by side	6–8
3	in a circle	8–10
4	in a circle	10–12
5	in a circle	15–20

Rice and Pasta

Like potatoes, rice and pasta are high in starchy carbohydrates. Both brown rice and whole grain pasta provide higher vitamin and mineral levels as well as fibre. Rice and pastas come in sufficient variety to delight the most adventurous cook and are economical food choices. Preparation of both is fast and easy. Just follow directions on the package.

Rice or Pasta on Call

We think having "rice on call" in the freezer is the ultimate home convenience food. You may well ask what is it? It is simply cooking extra rice, then measuring it into small freezer bags in appropriate serving sizes. Seal, label the bags and pop them into the freezer. Rice will keep frozen for up to six months. Keep "pasta on call" in the same manner as rice.

To Reheat Frozen Rice or Pasta

Rice: Remove rice from bag to small dish; add 1 tbsp (15 mL) water, cover with waxed paper and reheat on High (100%) for about 1 minute or until hot. Reheated rice makes a snap of Dinner menus #7, #11 and #26.

Pasta: Remove pasta from plastic bag; lower into small saucepan of boiling water. Return to boil and cook for 1 minute; drain. It is so convenient. (See Dinner menu #6.)

Protein Foods

Protein is the basic building material of life. It provides us with the amino acid building blocks we need for growth and repair of our bodies. Nine of these amino acids are called essential. They must come from our daily diet because our bodies cannot make them. All animal sources of protein are *complete* proteins because they contain all the nine essential amino acids.

Soybeans and quinoa are the only *complete* plant proteins. Other plant proteins are *incomplete* because they lack one or more of the nine essential amino acids. We can make them complete by combining plant proteins with one another. A general guide is to combine grains or nuts and seeds with legumes. And you don't have to combine complementary proteins at the same meal, as long as you are sure to eat a variety of sources over each day. Obviously, we must have sufficient and well-chosen forms of protein in our meals if we are to achieve a healthy lifestyle. (See Meat Alternatives below.)

We have focused on a wide variety of protein foods in our dinner menus. Some are vegetarian, some have chicken or meat, some fish or seafood. But they all provide about 3 PROTEIN CHOICES or 21 grams of protein in each dinner.

Is Meat a Healthy Food?

The saturated fat found in meat is its one downside and a reason for limiting the amount eaten. However, choosing leaner cuts of meat and trimming them well reduces this problem. Meat is exceptionally rich in iron, zinc and vitamins B6 and B12, as well as providing all nine of the essential amino acids.

Buying and Cooking Chicken, Meat and Fish

Since chicken, meat and fish are sold in grams, we have given metric weights in each menu and recipe. This will help you buy just the right amount when you are shopping. The size of each serving is based on the 100-gram portion recommended for healthy eating, often compared to the size of a deck of playing cards.

Our goal in cooking these foods is to suggest the quickest and most convenient method consistent with obtaining maximum flavour, tenderness and ease of digestion. In keeping with the advice of Canada's Food Guide to Healthy Eating to reduce total fat, we always advise the cooking method that uses the least fat.

Cooking meat successfully requires careful timing and temperature control. Some methods use gentle heat, some higher heat, but all methods conserve nutrients. Take beef as an example. Less tender cuts benefit from braising or stewing (see **Oven Beef Stew with Vegetables**, page 153). More tender cuts can be roasted, broiled or barbecued. Microwave cooking is preferred for reheating rather than primary cooking for meat and poultry. But for cooking fish, the microwave is excellent.

Meat Alternatives

The term "meat alternatives," according to Canada's Food Guide to Healthy Eating, refers to eggs, dairy products, legumes, grains, nuts and seeds. You don't always need meat or poultry to get the protein you require. It's possible to get all necessary nutrients from a vegetarian diet, especially if you include low-fat dairy products and/or eggs as in our **Baked Eggs with Tomato** (page 152) and **Three-Cheese Vegetarian Lasagna** (page 132). **Vegetable Spaghetti Sauce** (page 129), is another favourite. Total vegetarians (vegans) balance grains with legumes and seeds to obtain adequate protein. This can be difficult to manage with the carbohydrate restrictions of diabetes and needs expert knowledge and assistance.

Supermarket Meals

In a hurry or want a break from cooking? Your local supermarket offers many frozen chicken, meat, fish or pasta entrées in single-serving sizes. Although many are high in sodium, they are fine for occasional use. They can be conveniently heated and combined with vegetables and a salad for a satisfying meal. Just remember when shopping for frozen entrées to read labels carefully and compare. Look first at the amount of protein in one serving and then the amount of fat and calories. Choose the frozen entrée with the least fat and calories and the most protein. Compare the packaged entrées to our dinner menus, which contain about 20 grams of protein, a maximum of 15 grams of fat, about 60 grams of carbohydrate and around 500 calories for an *entire meal*, not just one course. See www.healthyeatingisinstore.ca for help in using labels.

Desserts

Canada's Food Guide to Healthy Eating recommends including more fruits in a greater variety in our meals. Well, our menus do just that. Fruit makes an excellent dessert. It tastes sweet, is relatively low in calories and often high in water content. Fruit is a major source of fibre, minerals and vitamins. Strawberries, pears and apples contain soluble fibre. Cantaloupe, oranges and bananas are rich in potassium. Most fruits are available all year long and the nice thing is that you can buy just one or two pieces at a time. And if you don't happen to have the fruit on hand suggested in a menu, check Appendix 2, page 227, for other fruit choices.

We use fruit in some great-tasting and easy dessert recipes. Consider **Jellied Fruit Parfait** (page 123) and **Pear Hélène** (page 126). **Homestyle Gingerbread with Warm Peach Sauce** (page 121) and **Fast and Healthy Apple Crisp** (page 145) are definitely favourite "comfort foods."

Meal Planning

You probably are getting the message by now. If you are serious about healthy eating, weight loss and diabetes control, you will plan to have three balanced meals every day. This means a good breakfast, a moderate-size lunch and not too large an evening meal (as well as whatever snacks you choose).

We have tried to include in our dinner menus many of your favourite comfort foods, updated to be lower in fat and calories. An occasional higher fat dessert has been balanced against a low-fat main course.

dinner menus

Each dinner menu provides about 500 calories* and is based on:

2 STARCH CHOICES
2 FRUITS & VEGETABLES CHOICES
1 MILK (1%) CHOICE
3 PROTEIN CHOICES
1 FATS & OILS CHOICE
1 EXTRA

*489 calories with skim milk, 499 calories with 1% milk
56 grams carbohydrate

dinner menu #1

3 slices (90 g) lean roast beef with horseradish
1/4 cup (50 mL) **Light Gravy** (page 119)

1 serving (1/4) **Oven-Roasted Winter Vegetables** (page 120)

1/2 cup (125 mL) green beans

1 serving (1/12) **Homestyle Gingerbread** (page 121)
with 1/3 cup (75 mL) **Warm Peach Sauce** (page 122)

tea or coffee with milk

dinner menu #2

3 thin slices (90 g) lean roast pork loin
with 1/4 cup (50 mL) unsweetened applesauce

1 medium (190 g) baked potato

1/2 cup (125 mL) mashed turnip

1 cup (250 mL) cooked spinach with 1 tsp (5 mL) soft margarine OR butter

1 serving (1/4) **Jellied Fruit Parfait** (page 123)

tea or coffee with milk

dinner menu #3

2 slices (60 g) cooked cold roast beef

1/2 cup (125 mL) **Summertime Potato Salad** (page 124)

1 small (30 g) dinner roll with 1 tsp (5 mL) soft margarine OR butter

celery sticks, dill pickle, tomato and cucumber slices

1 cup (250 mL) sweet black cherries

1/2 cup (125 mL) low-fat milk

tea or coffee

dinner menu #4

1 slice (1/6) **Baked Vegetable Meat Loaf** (page 125)

1/2 small baked acorn squash
10 steamed snow peas

1 serving (1/4) **Pear Hélène** (page 126)

tea or coffee with milk

dinner menu #5

1 serving (1/4) **Baked Fish and Vegetables en Papillote** (page 127)

1 cup (250 mL) cooked rice

sliced tomato and cucumber
with 1 tbsp (15 mL) **Herb Vinaigrette** (page 128)
OR 1 tbsp (15 mL) low-calorie Italian dressing

1 cup (250 mL) strawberries

1/2 cup (125 mL) low-fat milk

tea or coffee

dinner menu #6

1 cup (250 mL) **Vegetable Spaghetti Sauce** (page 129)
with 1 cup (250 mL) cooked spaghetti and 3 tbsp (45 mL) grated
Parmesan cheese

tossed salad with wedges of 1 hard-cooked egg
and 1 tbsp (15 mL) calorie-reduced Italian dressing

1/2 grapefruit, sprinkled with cinnamon and broiled

1/2 cup (125 mL) low-fat milk
tea or coffee

dinner menu #7

1 serving (1/4) **Oriental Chicken Stir-Fry** (page 130)
with 1 cup (250 mL) cooked rice

Raspberry Sundae
*1/4 cup (50 mL) unsweetened frozen raspberries over
1/3 cup (75 mL) light vanilla ice cream*

1/2 cup (125 mL) low-fat milk
tea or coffee

dinner menu #8

1 serving (1/5) **Provençale Chicken and Rice Dinner** (page 131)

1 cup (250 mL) steamed broccoli with lemon wedge

1 serving (1/4) **Microwave Applesauce** (page 75)

1/2 cup (125 mL) low-fat milk
tea or coffee

dinner menu #9
Informal Dinner for Six

1 serving (1/6) **Three-Cheese Vegetarian Lasagna** (page 132)

1 serving (1/6) **Favourite Caesar Salad** (page 133)

1/2 cup (125 mL) chilled cantaloupe cubes, 1/4 cup (50 mL) blueberries
with lime juice and rum extract

1/2 cup (125 mL) low-fat milk
tea or coffee

dinner menu #10

1 sole fillet (100 g) raw, baked or microwaved
with herbs, lemon juice and 1 tsp (5 mL) margarine OR butter

1 medium (190 g) boiled potato,
with parsley and 1 tsp (5 mL) soft margarine OR butter

1 serving (1/4) **Tomato Zucchini Bake** (page 134)

Ice Cream Sundae
*1/3 cup (75 mL) light ice cream with 1 tbsp (15 mL)
no-sugar-added fruit spread*

1/2 cup (125 mL) low-fat milk
tea or coffee

dinner menu #11
Saturday Night Supper

1 1/4 cups (300 mL) **Chili con Carne** (page 135)
with 1/2 cup (125 mL) cooked rice

1 serving (1/4) **Cabbage Waldorf Salad** (page 72)

1 small (30 g) whole wheat dinner roll with 1 tsp (5 mL)
soft margarine OR butter

1/2 cup (125 mL) low-fat milk
tea or coffee

dinner menu #12

1 serving (1/4) **Herbed Citrus Pork Chop** (page 136)

1 medium (190 g) microwave-baked sweet potato

1/2 cup (125 mL) steamed Brussel sprouts
with 1 tbsp (15 mL) walnuts, toasted and chopped
and 1/2 tsp (2 mL) soft margarine OR butter

1/2 cup (125 mL) unsweetened applesauce
1 chocolate-coated digestive cookie

tea or coffee with milk

dinner menu #13

Take-Out Night

1/4 skinless roaster chicken, white meat only, with seasoned sauce

1/2 large baked potato with 2 tbsp (25 mL) light sour cream

1 small roll with 1 tsp (5 mL) soft margarine OR butter

chef's salad
with 1 tbsp (15 mL) calorie-reduced salad dressing

diet soft drink

dinner menu #14

1 serving (1/4) **Broiled Rainbow Trout with Tomato** (page 137)

2 new potatoes (150 g) with parsley

6 steamed asparagus spears with lemon

1 serving (1/8) **Apple Bavarian Torte** (page 138)

tea or coffee with milk

dinner menu #15

1 serving (1/6) **Old-Fashioned Turkey Pot Pie** (page 139)

1 cup (250 mL) **Dilled Carrot Slaw** (page 140)

1/3 cup (75 mL) canned sliced pears in juice

2 **Oatmeal and Date Bars** (page 141)

tea or coffee with milk

dinner menu #16

1 1/3 cups (325 mL) **Hearty Lamb Scotch Broth** (page 142)

1 small crusty whole wheat roll (30 g)
with 1 tsp (5 mL) soft margarine OR butter

2/3 cup (150 mL) honeydew melon cubes,
1 tsp (5 mL) fresh lime juice and sweetener to taste

1/2 cup (125 mL) low-fat milk
tea or coffee

dinner menu #17

1 serving (1/4) **Double Cheese 'n Ham Casserole** (page 143)

tossed greens with 1 tbsp (15 mL) calorie-reduced Italian dressing

2 slices **Warm Garlic Bread** (page 144)

1 serving (1/4) **Fast and Healthy Apple Crisp** (page 145)

tea or coffee with milk

dinner menu #18

1 serving (1/4) **Asian Grilled Pork Tenderloin** (page 146)

2/3 cup (150 mL) cooked brown rice with sliced green onion

1 serving (1/4) **Vegetable Kebabs** (page 147)

2/3 cup (150 mL) sliced mango
with 1/4 cup (50 mL) low-fat French vanilla yogurt with aspartame

tea or coffee with milk

dinner menu #19

1 grilled hamburger patty (1/2 cup/125 mL) lean ground beef
1 hamburger bun (60 g) with choice of toppings
(mustard, lettuce, tomatoes and onions, sliced)

6 raw mini carrots and cucumber slices

1/4 small cantaloupe with 1/3 cup (75 mL) light vanilla ice cream

tea or coffee with milk

dinner menu #20

1 serving (1/4) **Calves' Liver with Onion and Herbs** (page 148)

1 small (95 g) potato

1/2 cup (125 mL) green beans
with 1 tbsp (15 mL) chopped red pepper and lemon wedge

1 medium baked apple (150 g raw), with cinnamon
topped with 1 tbsp (15 mL) light sour cream

1/2 cup (125 mL) low-fat milk
tea or coffee

dinner menu #21

1 serving **Spanish Omelette** (page 149)

1 toasted English muffin (60 g)

1/2 cup (125 mL) light vanilla ice cream
with 1/2 cup (125 mL) sliced peaches

1/2 cup (125 mL) low-fat milk
tea or coffee

dinner menu #22

1 serving (1/2) **Crispy Chicken Fingers**
with **Creamy Dipping Sauce** (page 150)

1 cup cooked broccoli with 1 tsp (5 mL) soft margarine OR butter

1 serving (1/2) **Baked Sliced Apples** (page 151)

tea or coffee with milk

dinner menu #23

1 serving (1/2) **Baked Eggs with Tomato** (page 152)

1 stalk steamed broccoli

1 small banana

1/2 cup (125 mL) low-fat milk
tea or coffee

dinner menu #24

1 cup (250 mL) **Oven Beef Stew with Vegetables** (page 153)

1 small (95 g) boiled potato

1/2 cup (125 mL) steamed snow peas with
1 tsp (5 mL) soft margarine OR butter

1/4 cantaloupe wedge with lime

1/2 cup (125 mL) low-fat milk
tea or coffee

dinner menu #25

1 ham slice (120 g) with 1 tsp (5 mL) Dijon mustard

1/2 cup (125 mL) green peas with
2 sliced mushrooms and 1/2 tsp (2 mL) soft margarine OR butter

1 serving (1/2) **Scalloped Sweet and White Potatoes** (page 154)

1 serving (1/4) **Pineapple Smoothie Dessert** (page 155)

tea or coffee with milk

dinner menu #26

1 serving (1/2) **Mushroom Seafood Strogonoff** (page 156)

1/2 cup (125 mL) cooked rice

6 steamed asparagus spears with lemon

1/2 cup (125 mL) light vanilla ice cream with 1/2 cup (125 mL) raspberries

tea or coffee with milk

dinner menu #27

1 serving (1/2) **Veal Cutlets in Tomato Herb Sauce** (page 157)

1/2 small cooked acorn squash with 1 tsp (5 mL) soft margarine OR butter

1 crusty roll (30 g) with 1 tsp (5 mL) soft margarine OR butter

1/2 small banana, sliced, over low-calorie jellied dessert

1/2 cup (125 mL) low-fat milk
tea or coffee

dinner menu #28

1 serving (1/2) **Baked Whitefish** (page 158)

1/2 cup (125 mL) cooked sliced carrots

1 stalk steamed broccoli

1 serving (1/2) **Rosemary Roasted Potatoes** (page 159)

1 serving (1/4) **Light Lemon Mousse** (page 160)
2 ginger snap cookies

1/2 cup (125 mL) low-fat milk
tea or coffee

dinner menu #29

1 serving (1/2) **Herbed Chicken and Vegetables** (page 161)
over 2/3 cup (150 mL) cooked brown rice

1 cup (250 mL) torn spinach
with 1 tbsp (15 mL) **Warm Sherry Vinaigrette** (page 162)

1 serving (1/3) **Raspberry Cream Dessert** (page 163)

tea or coffee with milk

dinner menu #30

Holiday Dinner

2 slices (60 g) **Roast Turkey Breast**
with 1/2 cup (125 mL) **Stuffing** (page 164)

1/4 cup (50 mL) **Light Gravy** (page 119)

2 tbsp (25 mL) **Light Cranberry Sauce** (page 165)

1/2 cup (125 mL) mashed potatoes with milk

1/2 cup (125 mL) cooked green peas

1/2 cup (125 mL) light chocolate ice cream

tea or coffee with milk

dinner recipes index

dinner menus #1, #30

Light Gravy

To make perfect low-fat gravy for roast chicken, turkey or beef, prepare with pan drippings that have all visible fat removed.

	Pan juices	
	Water or vegetable liquid	
2 tbsp	cornstarch	25 mL
	Salt and freshly ground pepper	

1 Pour pan juices through sieve into 2 cup (500 mL) measuring cup. Skim fat with spoon or bulb baster; or drop ice cubes into strained pan juices to chill fat layer; remove hardened fat with ice.

2 Add enough water or vegetable liquid to pan juices to measure 1 1/2 cups (375 mL). Return to roasting pan; bring to boil.

3 Mix cornstarch with 2 tbsp (25 mL) cold water. Gradually add to boiling liquid; cook and stir for 5 minutes or until smooth and thickened. Season to taste with salt and pepper.

Makes 6 servings, 1 1/2 cups (375 mL).

PREPARATION TIME:
10 minutes

COOKING TIME:
about 8 minutes

Each serving:
1/4 cup (50 mL)

1 EXTRA

3 g carbohydrate (0 g fibre)
1 g protein
0 g total fat
195 mg sodium
15 calories

PREPARATION TIME:
15 minutes

COOKING TIME:
1 hour

Each serving:
1/4 of recipe

1/2 STARCH CHOICE
1 1/2 FRUITS & VEGETABLES
CHOICES
1 FATS & OILS CHOICE

27 g carbohydrate (5 g fibre)
3 g protein
3 g total fat (1 g saturated fat)
90 mg sodium
155 calories

KITCHEN TIP

These root vegetables all cook in about the same amount of time. Cut vegetable pieces in a similar size for even baking.

dinner menu #1
Oven-Roasted Winter Vegetables

Northern climate cooks have always been challenged to develop superb-tasting root vegetable dishes. This recipe meets the challenge. One serving is an excellent source of vitamin A and is high in fibre.

1	medium parsnip, cut into 8 large pieces (see Tip) (1 1/2 cups/375 mL)	1
8	turnip pieces (1 1/2 cups/375 mL)	8
8	peeled potato pieces, (1 medium)	8
2	medium carrots, cut into 12 chunks	2
2	medium onions, quartered	2
1 tbsp	melted soft margarine OR butter	15 mL
2 tbsp	dark rum OR 1 tsp (5 mL) rum extract	25 mL
1/2 tsp	ground nutmeg	2 mL
Pinch	each: salt and freshly ground pepper	Pinch

1 In shallow casserole, place parsnip, turnip, potato, carrots and onions. Combine margarine, rum, nutmeg, salt and pepper. Drizzle over vegetables.

2 Cover and bake in 350°F (180°C) oven for 1 hour or until vegetables are tender.

Makes 4 servings.

dinner menu #1

150-calorie snack menu #18, 300-calorie snack menu #13

Homestyle Gingerbread

Homemade gingerbread with **Warm Peach Sauce** (see page 122) or plain yogurt—either way they are superb desserts. Or make the batter into a soft cookie (see page 122). **Multimix** (page 36) speeds the preparation!

Gingerbread Cake

2 cups	**Multimix** (page 36)	500 mL
2 tbsp	granulated sugar	25 mL
2 tsp	ground ginger	10 mL
1 tsp	ground cinnamon	5 mL
1 tsp	baking soda	5 mL
2/3 cup	boiling water	150 mL
1/4 cup	fancy molasses	50 mL
1	egg, beaten	1

1 In large bowl, combine **Multimix**, sugar, ginger, cinnamon and baking soda.

2 Stir boiling water, molasses and egg into dry ingredients just until moistened.

3 Spoon batter into lightly greased 8-inch (2 L) square baking pan. Bake in 350°F (180°C) oven for 35 minutes or until top springs back when lightly touched. Serve warm.

Makes 12 servings.

PREPARATION TIME:
10 minutes

COOKING TIME:
35 minutes

Each serving:
1/12 of recipe

1 STARCH CHOICE
1 FATS & OILS CHOICE

16 g carbohydrate (1 g fibre)
2 g protein
5 g total fat (1 g saturated fat)
307 mg sodium
116 calories

Soft Ginger Currant Cookie

1 Add 1/4 cup (50 mL) dried currants to **Homestyle Gingerbread** batter (see page 121) and drop as a soft cookie onto a baking sheet lightly sprayed with nonstick cooking spray. Bake in 350°F (180°C) oven for 8 to 10 minutes.

Makes 24 soft cookies.

Each serving:
2 cookies

1/2 STARCH CHOICE
1/2 FRUITS & VEGETABLES CHOICE
1/2 SUGARS CHOICE
1 FATS & OILS CHOICE

19 g carbohydrate (1 g fibre)
2 g protein
5 g total fat (1 g saturated fat)
149 mg sodium
124 calories

dinner menu #1
Warm Peach Sauce

Peach and citrus flavours make this warm sauce the perfect accompaniment to our **Homestyle Gingerbread** (see page 121).

1 cup	fresh or frozen sliced peaches	250 mL
1/3 cup	orange juice	75 mL
1 tbsp	lemon juice	15 mL
2 tsp	brown sugar	10 mL
Pinch	ground nutmeg	Pinch

PREPARATION TIME:
5 minutes

COOKING TIME:
5 minutes

Each serving:
1/3 cup (75 mL)

1 FRUITS & VEGETABLES CHOICE

12 g carbohydrate (1 g fibre)
1 g protein
0 g total fat
3 mg sodium
48 calories

1 In small saucepan, combine peaches, orange and lemon juice, sugar and nutmeg. Cook, covered, over low heat for 5 minutes or until peaches are tender. Remove from heat, mash peaches slightly and serve sauce warm.

Makes 4 servings, 1 1/3 cups (325 mL).

dinner menu #2

Jellied Fruit Parfait

Crushed pineapple and yogurt in fruit-flavoured gelatin make an eye-catching light dessert.

1	pkg (10.2 g) fruit-flavoured light jelly powder	1
1 cup	boiling water	250 mL
1 cup	cold water	250 mL
3/4 cup	crushed pineapple	175 mL
2 cups	low-calorie (1%) plain yogurt	500 mL

1 Place jelly powder in medium bowl. Stir in boiling water until completely dissolved. Stir in cold water. Cover and refrigerate until set.

2 For each serving:
Layer 1/2 cup (125 mL) jelly with 3 tbsp (45 mL) pineapple and 1/2 cup (125 mL) yogurt, alternating layers more than once if desired.

Makes 4 servings.

PREPARATION TIME:
10 minutes

CHILL:
45 minutes

Each serving:
1/4 of recipe

1 FRUITS & VEGETABLES CHOICE
1 MILK 1% CHOICE
1/2 PROTEIN CHOICE

16 g carbohydrate (1 g fibre)
9 g protein
2 g total fat (1 g saturated fat)
145 mg sodium
115 calories

PREPARATION TIME:
30 minutes

CHILL:
30 minutes or longer

Each serving:
1/2 cup (125 mL)

1 STARCH CHOICE
1 FATS & OILS CHOICE

16 g carbohydrate (1 g fibre)
4 g protein
4 g total fat (1 g saturated fat)
293 mg sodium
115 calories

dinner menu #3
special occasions menu #5

Summertime Potato Salad

When the weather outside is steamy, carefree cool meals are important. Prepare this chilled salad ahead of time.

3	medium potatoes, cubed (2 1/3 cups/575 mL)	3
2	eggs	2
2/3 cup	sliced celery	150 mL
1/4 cup	sliced green onion	50 mL
1/4 cup	chopped parsley	50 mL
1/4 cup	light mayonnaise	50 mL
1/4 cup	low-fat (1%) plain yogurt	50 mL
1 tbsp	malt vinegar	15 mL
1/2 tsp	each: salt and dried tarragon	2 mL
1/4 tsp	dry mustard	1 mL
1/4 tsp	freshly ground pepper	1 mL
	Leaf lettuce	

1 In saucepan, cook potatoes in boiling water for 10 minutes or until just tender; drain and cool. Simmer eggs in water in separate saucepan for 20 minutes. Drain well and cool. Peel and cut eggs into quarters; set aside.

2 Combine potatoes, celery, onion and parsley. Stir together mayonnaise, yogurt, vinegar, salt, tarragon, mustard and pepper. Stir gently into potato mixture. Place in a bowl lined with lettuce leaves and garnish with egg quarters. Cover and chill until serving time.

Makes 7 servings, 3 1/2 cups (875 mL) salad.

dinner menu #4

Baked Vegetable Meat Loaf

Vegetables add special extra flavour and moisture to this comfort-food favourite.

1 lb	lean ground beef	500 g
1/2 cup	rolled oats	125 mL
1/3 cup	finely chopped carrot	75 mL
1/3 cup	finely chopped celery	75 mL
3 tbsp	finely chopped onion	45 mL
3 tbsp	chopped parsley	45 mL
1/2 cup	tomato sauce	125 mL
1	egg, lightly beaten	1
2 tsp	prepared mustard	10 mL
1/4 tsp	salt	1 mL
1/4 tsp	freshly ground pepper	1 mL
1/4 tsp	chili powder	1 mL

1 Spray 9 × 5-inch (2 L) loaf pan with nonstick coating.

2 In large bowl, combine beef, rolled oats, carrot, celery, onion and parsley; mix well.

3 Combine tomato sauce, egg, mustard, salt, pepper and chili powder. Lightly combine meat mixture with tomato mixture just until mixed. Turn into loaf pan.

4 Bake in 375°F (190°C) oven for 50 minutes or until meat is cooked. Drain off any fat. Allow to stand for 5 minutes before cutting into 6 slices.

Makes 6 servings.

PREPARATION TIME:
20 minutes

COOKING TIME:
50 minutes

Each serving:
1 slice

1/2 STARCH CHOICE
2 1/2 PROTEIN CHOICES

8 g carbohydrate (2 g fibre)
17 g protein
10 g total fat (4 g saturated fat)
281 mg sodium
187 calories

PREPARATION TIME:
15 minutes

COOKING TIME:
about 5 minutes

Each serving:
1/4 of recipe

1/2 STARCH CHOICE
1 FRUITS & VEGETABLES CHOICE
1 MILK 2% CHOICE

23 g carbohydrate (1 g fibre)
5 g protein
3 g total fat (1 g saturated fat)
443 mg sodium
130 calories

dinner menu #4
Pear Hélène

Although not an authentic version of the original classic dessert, our much easier-to-make version is still delicious.

1	pkg (40 g) light instant chocolate pudding with aspartame	1
2 cups	low-fat milk	500 mL
4	pear halves, canned in juice, drained	4

1 Prepare chocolate pudding according to package directions. Cover and refrigerate for 1 hour or until cool.

2 Place one pear half in each of four bowls. Spoon one-quarter of pudding over each pear.

Makes 4 servings.

dinner menu #5

Baked Fish and Vegetables en Papillote

En papillote means steaming in parchment paper or aluminum foil. It is a fast and healthy way to bake a meal in a package. Choose fish that can be cut into fairly thick pieces, for example, turbot, halibut or haddock.

3/4 lb	fresh OR frozen and thawed fish	375 g
1/2 cup	finely chopped carrot (1 medium)	125 mL
4	large mushrooms, sliced	4
1	green onion, chopped	1
1/4 cup	chopped parsley	50 mL
1 tbsp	lemon juice	15 mL
1 tbsp	melted soft margarine OR butter	15 mL
1/2 tsp	dried thyme	2 mL
	Salt and pepper to taste	

PREPARATION TIME:
15 minutes

COOKING TIME:
20 minutes

Each serving:
1/4 of recipe

3 PROTEIN CHOICES
1 EXTRA

3 g carbohydrate (1 g fibre)
20 g protein
4 g total fat (1 g saturated fat)
129 mg sodium
131 calories

1 Cut four sheets of parchment paper or aluminum foil into squares 2 inches (5 cm) larger than fish fillets. Spray paper or foil with nonstick vegetable coating. Cut fish into four equal-size pieces; place in centre of paper or foil.

2 Distribute carrot, mushrooms and onion evenly over fish.

3 Combine parsley, lemon juice, margarine, thyme, salt and pepper. Spoon over vegetables. Fold long ends of paper or foil twice so fish is tightly enclosed. Lift short ends, bring together and fold twice. Place on baking pan.

4 Bake in 400°F (200°C) oven 20 minutes or until fish flakes easily with a fork and vegetables are tender. Place packages on dinner plates for each person to open at the table.

Makes 4 servings.

PREPARATION TIME:
10 minutes

CHILL:
up to two weeks

Each serving:
2 tbsp (25 mL)

1 FATS & OILS CHOICE

1 g carbohydrate (0 g fibre)
0 g protein
5 g total fat (0 g saturated fat)
215 mg sodium
46 calories

KITCHEN TIP

Use this dressing as a marinade for chicken, beef and pork as well as vegetables.

Use about 1/3 cup (75 mL) dressing to marinate each 1 lb (500 g) of meat.

Herb Vinaigrette Dressing

Here's a zesty dressing to serve with leafy green salads or to drizzle over sliced cucumbers and tomatoes. And it doubles as a flavourful and tenderizing marinade for barbecuing meat (see Tip). Truly versatile!

1/4 cup	red wine vinegar	50 mL
1/4 cup	chicken stock	50 mL
2 tbsp	lemon OR lime juice	25 mL
1 tsp	dried tarragon, optional	5 mL
1/2 tsp	dry mustard	2 mL
1/2 tsp	paprika	2 mL
1/2 tsp	garlic salt	2 mL
1/4 tsp	freshly ground pepper	1 mL
Dash	hot pepper sauce	Dash
2 tbsp	olive oil	25 mL

1 In container with a tight-fitting lid, combine vinegar, chicken stock, lemon juice, tarragon, mustard, paprika, garlic salt, pepper and hot pepper sauce; shake well. Add oil and shake again. Refrigerate for up to two weeks.

Makes 3/4 cup (175 mL).

dinner menus #6 and #9

Vegetable Spaghetti Sauce

You'll be amazed at the many uses you'll find for this inexpensive vegetarian sauce. Use it for lasagna (see Tip), as a sauce over chicken or with ground beef as a traditional sauce for spaghetti.

1 tbsp	canola oil	15 mL
3 cups	finely chopped zucchini (3 medium)	750 mL
1 cup	chopped onion (1 medium)	250 mL
1/2 cup	finely chopped carrot (1 medium)	125 mL
2	cloves garlic, minced	2
1	can (28 oz/798 mL) tomatoes	1
1	can (7.5 oz/213 mL) tomato sauce	1
1	can (10 oz/284 mL) mushroom stems and pieces	1
2 tsp	dried oregano	10 mL
1 1/2 tsp	dried basil	7 mL
1 tsp	salt	5 mL
1/4 tsp	pepper	1 mL

1 In large saucepan, heat oil over medium-high heat. Add zucchini, onion, carrot and garlic. Cook for 10 minutes or until onions are tender; stir frequently. Break up tomatoes. Add tomatoes and liquid, tomato sauce, mushrooms and liquid, oregano, basil, salt and pepper. Cover and simmer for 2 hours or until sauce is thickened; stir occasionally.

Makes 6 servings, 6 cups (1.5 L) sauce.

PREPARATION TIME:
20 minutes

COOKING TIME:
2 hours

Each serving:
1 cup (250 mL)

1 FRUITS & VEGETABLES CHOICE
1 FATS & OILS CHOICE

15 g carbohydrate (4 g fibre)
3 g protein
3 g total fat (0 g saturated fat)
952 mg sodium
88 calories

KITCHEN TIP

Double the recipe and freeze **Vegetable Spaghetti Sauce** in amounts of 4 cups (1 L) for **Three-Cheese Vegetarian Lasagna** (page 132)

PREPARATION TIME:
20 minutes

COOKING TIME:
11 minutes for stir-fry

Each serving:
1/4 of recipe

1/2 FRUITS & VEGETABLES CHOICE
3 PROTEIN CHOICES
1 EXTRA

8 g carbohydrate (2 g fibre)
22 g protein
6 g total fat (1 g saturated fat)
828 mg sodium
174 calories

KITCHEN TIP

Use **Homemade Chicken Broth** (page 91) or chicken broth from chicken bouillon cubes or sachets prepared to package directions.

dinner menu #7
Oriental Chicken Stir-fry

Stir-fry recipes provide a delicious way of adding lots of vegetables to a small amount of meat.

1 tbsp	canola oil	15 mL
3/4 lb	boneless chicken breast, cut into thin strips	375 g
2 cups	broccoli florets	500 mL
2/3 cup	chopped red pepper	150 mL
3	green onions, diagonally sliced	3
1	clove garlic, minced	1
2 cups	sliced mushrooms	500 mL
1 cup	sliced celery	250 mL
1/2 cup	chicken broth (see Tip)	125 mL
1 tbsp	cornstarch	15 mL
2 tsp	soy sauce	10 mL
1/2 tsp	ground ginger	2 mL

1 In wok or large nonstick skillet, heat oil over high heat. Add chicken; cook for 3 minutes, stirring constantly.

2 Add broccoli, red pepper, onions and garlic; cover and steam for 5 minutes. Add mushrooms and celery; cover and steam for 2 minutes.

3 Combine chicken broth, cornstarch, soy sauce and ginger; pour over chicken mixture. Stir-fry for 1 minute, or until sauce thickens.

Makes 4 servings.

dinner menu #8

Provençale Chicken and Rice Dinner

Ultimate convenience in meal preparation must be the "meal in a dish." Chicken in combination with rice and vegetables makes this an easily prepared meal.

5	large chicken thighs (1 1/2 lb/750 g) (see Tip)	5
1/2 tsp	salt	2 mL
1/4 tsp	pepper	1 mL

Vegetable-Rice

1/2 cup	chopped onion (1 small)	125 mL
1/2 cup	chopped green pepper	125 mL
1/4 cup	water	50 mL
1	can (28 oz/798 mL) tomatoes	1
3/4 cup	uncooked long grain rice	175 mL
1 tsp	garlic powder	5 mL

1 Remove and discard skin and fat from chicken. Sprinkle chicken with salt and pepper. In large nonstick skillet, brown chicken over medium heat on both sides. Remove to deep 6 cup (1.5 L) casserole.

2 In same skillet, cook onion and green pepper in water for 5 minutes. Chop tomatoes; combine undrained tomatoes with vegetables, rice and garlic powder. Spoon over meat in casserole. Cover and bake in 325°F (160°C) oven for 1 1/4 hours or until liquid is absorbed and rice is cooked.

Makes 5 servings, 5 chicken thighs and 5 cups (1.25 L) vegetable-rice.

PREPARATION TIME:
20 minutes

COOKING TIME:
1 1/4 hours

Each serving:
1 chicken thigh and 1 cup (250 mL) vegetable-rice

1 1/2 STARCH CHOICES
1/2 FRUITS & VEGETABLES CHOICE
3 PROTEIN CHOICES

31 g carbohydrate (2 g fibre)
24 g protein
7 g total fat (2 g saturated fat)
879 mg sodium
283 calories

KITCHEN TIP

Chicken may be replaced with 5 lean boneless pork chops (100 g each) cut 1/2 inch (1 cm) thick.

PREPARATION TIME:
20 minutes (if **Vegetable Spaghetti Sauce** is prepared.)

COOKING TIME:
60 minutes

Each serving:
1/6 of recipe

1 1/2 STARCH CHOICES
1 FRUITS & VEGETABLES CHOICE
3 PROTEIN CHOICES

36 g carbohydrate (6 g fibre)
26 g protein
9 g total fat (0 g saturated fat)
1389 mg sodium
325 calories

dinner menu #9
Three-Cheese Vegetarian Lasagna

This vegetarian high-fibre version of lasagna uses our **Vegetable Spaghetti Sauce** (see page 129) along with vegetables and three cheeses.

8	lasagna noodles	8
2	pkgs (300 g) frozen chopped spinach, thawed and well drained	2
1	carton (500 g) low-fat (1%) cottage cheese	1
1	egg	1
1/2 tsp	salt	2 mL
1/4 tsp	freshly ground pepper	1 mL
1/4 tsp	ground nutmeg	1 mL
4 cups	**Vegetable Spaghetti Sauce** (page 129)	1 L
1 1/2 cups	shredded low-fat mozzarella cheese	375 mL
2 tbsp	grated Parmesan cheese	25 mL

1 In large pot of boiling water, cook lasagna according to package directions or until al dente (tender but firm). Drain well and set aside.

2 Combine spinach, cottage cheese, egg, salt, pepper and nutmeg.

3 Spread 1 cup (250 mL) spaghetti sauce in bottom of 13 × 9-inch (3.5 L) baking pan. Place 4 noodles, overlapping, over sauce; add one-half spinach mixture and one-half remaining spaghetti sauce; repeat layers. Sprinkle evenly with mozzarella and Parmesan cheeses.

4 Bake in 350°F (180°C) oven for 1 hour or until hot and bubbly; let stand 10 minutes before cutting.

Makes 6 servings.

dinner menu #9

special occasions menu #4

Favourite Caesar Salad

Enjoy this lower fat version of the famous Caesar salad. You'll have enough dressing for another meal.

Salad Dressing

3 tbsp	light mayonnaise	45 mL
1	clove garlic, minced	1
2 tbsp	red wine vinegar	25 mL
1 tbsp	Dijon mustard	15 mL
1 tbsp	lemon juice	15 mL
Dash	hot pepper sauce	Dash
Dash	Worcestershire sauce	Dash
1/4 cup	olive oil	50 mL
2 tbsp	water	25 mL

Salad

8 cups	torn romaine lettuce leaves (about 1 head)	2 L
1 1/2 cups	toasted bread croutons	375 mL
1 tbsp	grated Parmesan cheese	15 mL

1 Whisk together mayonnaise, garlic, vinegar, mustard, lemon juice, hot pepper sauce and Worcestershire sauce. Gradually whisk in olive oil and water until blended and smooth.

2 Place torn lettuce, croutons and cheese in large salad bowl. Toss with 1/3 cup (75 mL) salad dressing (about 1/2 of dressing). Refrigerate remaining dressing for a second salad.

Makes 6 servings and 2/3 cup (150 mL) salad dressing.

PREPARATION TIME:
15 minutes

Each serving:
1/6 of recipe

**1/2 STARCH CHOICE
2 FATS & OILS CHOICES**

9 g carbohydrate (**1 g fibre**)
2 g protein
8 g total fat (1 g saturated fat)
156 mg sodium
119 calories

KITCHEN TIP

For a single serving of salad, use about 1 cup (250 mL) torn romaine lettuce leaves, 1/4 cup (50 mL) toasted bread croutons, 1 tbsp (15 mL) salad dressing and 1/2 tsp (2 mL) grated Parmesan cheese.

PREPARATION TIME:
10 minutes

COOKING TIME:
15 minutes

Each serving:
1/4 of recipe

1/2 FRUITS & VEGETABLES CHOICE
1 EXTRA

5 g carbohydrate (2 g fibre)
2 g protein
1 g total fat (1 g saturated fat)
186 mg sodium
34 calories

dinner menu #10

Tomato Zucchini Bake

This easy-to-make recipe puts summer's garden vegetables to excellent use.

2	medium tomatoes, sliced	2
1	medium zucchini, thinly sliced	1
1	green onion, sliced	1
2 tbsp	grated Parmesan cheese	25 mL
1/4 tsp	salt	1 mL
1/4 tsp	freshly ground pepper	1 mL
1/4 tsp	dried oregano	1 mL

1 In a shallow casserole, layer tomato slices and zucchini in an overlapping circle. Top with green onion; sprinkle with cheese, salt, pepper and oregano.

2 Bake, uncovered, in 350°F (180°C) oven for 20 minutes or until vegetables are just tender.

Makes 4 servings.

dinner menu #11

Chili con Carne

Chili tucked away in the freezer is a gift from food heaven on a busy day. This recipe makes a large amount thanks to the addition of "extra" vegetables.

1 lb	lean ground beef	500 g
1 cup	chopped onion (1 medium)	250 mL
1	clove garlic, crushed	1
3 cups	finely shredded cabbage	750 mL
2 cups	thinly sliced celery	500 mL
1/2 cup	chopped green pepper (1/2 medium)	125 mL
1	can (28 oz/798 mL) tomatoes	1
1	can (7.5 oz/213 mL) tomato sauce	1
1	can (19 oz/540 mL) kidney beans, drained	1
1 tbsp	chili powder	15 mL
1 tsp	dried oregano	5 mL
1 tsp	salt	5 mL
1/4 tsp	hot pepper sauce	1 mL

1 In large nonstick skillet, cook beef over medium-high heat until brown and crumbly. Drain off fat. Add onion and garlic; cook for 5 minutes.

2 Add cabbage, celery, green pepper, tomatoes, tomato sauce, kidney beans, chili powder, oregano, salt and hot pepper sauce. Cover and simmer over medium-low heat for 45 minutes or until vegetables are tender; stir occasionally.

Makes about 8 servings, 9 cups (2.25 L).

PREPARATION TIME:
20 minutes

COOKING TIME:
about 45 minutes

Each serving:
1 1/4 cups (300 mL)

1 STARCH CHOICE
2 PROTEIN CHOICES

21 g carbohydrate (7 g fibre)
16 g protein
6 g total fat (2 g saturated fat)
835 mg sodium
195 calories

PREPARATION TIME:
10 minutes

COOKING TIME:
about 10 minutes

Each serving:
1/4 of recipe

**1/2 FRUITS & VEGETABLES
CHOICE
3 PROTEIN CHOICES**

3 g carbohydrate (0 g fibre)
22 g protein
6 g total fat (2 g saturated fat)
76 mg sodium
158 calories

Herbed Citrus Pork Chop

Citrus is a wonderful complement to pork in this very easy-to-make recipe.

4	boneless loin pork chops (each 100 g raw)	4
1/4 cup	orange juice	50 mL
1 tsp	Dijon mustard	5 mL
1 tsp	liquid honey	5 mL
1/4 tsp	each: dried thyme, tarragon, salt and freshly ground pepper	1 mL

1 Trim and discard fat from chops. In a large non-stick skillet, cook chops on medium for 5 minutes per side or until brown.

2 In small bowl, stir together orange juice, mustard, honey, thyme, tarragon, salt and pepper. Spoon sauce over chops. Cover and cook for 5 minutes or until chops are just cooked.

Makes 4 servings.

dinner menu #14

Broiled Rainbow Trout with Tomato

Broiling preserves the delicate texture and flavour of rainbow trout. One serving is an excellent source of niacin and B12.

1 lb	rainbow trout fillets (2 medium) OR 4 small (1/4 lb/125 g)	500 g
1/2 cup	finely chopped fresh cilantro	125 mL
2 tbsp	lime juice	25 mL
1 tsp	olive oil	5 mL
1/2 tsp	grated lime rind	2 mL
Pinch	each: salt and freshly ground pepper	Pinch
1/2 cup	chopped tomato	125 mL

1 Wipe fish with paper towelling; split fillets lengthwise. Spray shallow baking pan with nonstick vegetable coating; arrange fillets in single layer.

2 Stir together cilantro, juice, oil, rind, salt and pepper. Combine 2 tbsp (25 mL) with chopped tomato. Set aside.

3 Spread remainder of cilantro mixture over fish; allow to stand for 10 minutes.

4 Broil fish 4 inches (10 cm) from heat for 5 minutes or until fish is opaque and flakes easily.

5 Serve each one-half fillet with reserved tomato mixture.

Makes 4 servings.

PREPARATION TIME:
10 minutes

COOKING TIME:
5 minutes

Each serving:
1/2 fillet with 1/4 of tomato mixture

3 PROTEIN CHOICES
1 EXTRA

2 g carbohydrate (1 g fibre)
24 g protein
5 g total fat (1 g saturated fat)
144 mg sodium
153 calories

PREPARATION TIME:
30 minutes

COOKING TIME:
about 40 minutes

Each serving:
1/8 recipe

1/2 STARCH CHOICE
1 FRUITS & VEGETABLES CHOICE
1/2 SUGARS CHOICE
1/2 PROTEIN CHOICE
2 FATS & OILS CHOICES

23 g carbohydrate (1 g fibre)
6 g protein
10 g total fat (5 g saturated fat)
366 mg sodium
236 calories

1 **Crust**: Spray 9-inch (23 cm) springform pan with nonstick vegetable coating. Blend wafer crumbs, melted margarine and cinnamon. Press into bottom of pan. Bake in 350°F (180°C) oven for 8 minutes or until lightly browned.

2 **Filling**: In food processor or with electric mixer, blend cream cheese, egg whites, sweetener and vanilla until very smooth; spoon over crust.

dinner menu #14
Apple Bavarian Torte

This lower-fat version of the famous Bavarian dessert replaces the rich shortbread base with a wafer crumb crust.

Crust

1 cup	graham wafer crumbs (about 12 crackers)	250 mL
2 tbsp	melted soft margarine OR butter	25 mL
1/2 tsp	ground cinnamon	2 mL

Filling

1	pkg (250 g) light cream cheese	1
2	egg whites	2
1/4 cup	granular low-calorie sweetener with sucralose	50 mL
1 tsp	vanilla extract	5 mL
2 1/4 cups	peeled, cored and thinly sliced apples (2 medium apples)	550 mL
3 tbsp	packed brown sugar	45 mL
2 tbsp	soft margarine OR butter	25 mL
2 tbsp	all purpose flour	25 mL
1/2 tsp	ground cinnamon	2 mL
1/4 cup	slivered almonds	50 mL

3 Arrange apple slices in circles in single layer over cheese layer. In bowl, combine sugar, margarine, flour and cinnamon until coarse crumbs. Sprinkle over apples; top with almonds.

4 Bake in 350°F (180°C) oven for 45 minutes or until apples are tender. Cool and cut into 8 wedges.

Makes 8 servings.

dinner menu #15

Old-Fashioned Turkey Pot Pie

Generations of good cooks have been using their roasted chicken and turkey leftovers in a pot pie. This one is so good you may not want to wait for leftovers!

3 cups	skim milk	750 mL
1/3 cup	all purpose flour	75 mL
2 tbsp	Dijon mustard	25 mL
2	pkgs reduced-salt instant chicken bouillon	2
1 tsp	dried thyme leaves OR 2 tsp (10 mL) fresh	5 mL
1/4 tsp	each: paprika and freshly ground pepper	1 mL
1 tsp	soft margarine OR butter	5 mL
1 cup	sliced mushrooms	250 mL
4 cups	cubed cooked turkey OR chicken	1 L
1 1/2 cups	frozen peas	375 mL
1/3 cup	diced pimento	75 mL

Biscuit Topping

1 1/2 cups	**Multimix** (page 36)	375 mL
2 tbsp	chopped fresh parsley	25 mL
1/2 tsp	dried marjoram OR rosemary	2 mL
1/2 cup	skim milk	125 mL

1 In saucepan, whisk together milk, flour, mustard, bouillon, thyme, paprika and pepper. Bring slowly to a boil, stirring often. Reduce heat and simmer for 5 minutes or until smooth and thickened. Remove from heat.

PREPARATION TIME:
20 minutes

COOKING TIME:
45 minutes

Each serving:
1/6 of recipe with 1 biscuit

1 STARCH CHOICE
1 FRUITS & VEGETABLES CHOICE
1 MILK SKIM CHOICE
3 1/2 PROTEIN CHOICES

34 g carbohydrate (4 g fibre)
31 g protein
10 g total fat (3 g saturated fat)
540 mg sodium, 346 calories

2 In nonstick skillet, heat margarine on medium-high; cook mushrooms for 5 minutes or until golden. Stir mushrooms, turkey, peas and pimento into sauce. Turn into 6 cup (1.5 L) casserole.

3 **Biscuit Topping:** In small bowl, combine **Multimix**, parsley and marjoram. Stir in milk to form soft dough. Drop 6 large spoonfuls over turkey.

4 Bake in 375°F (190°C) oven for 45 minutes or until top is golden brown and biscuits are cooked.

Makes 6 servings.

PREPARATION TIME:
20 minutes

Each serving:
1 cup (250 mL)

1/2 FRUITS & VEGETABLES CHOICE
1 FATS & OILS CHOICE

8 g carbohydrate (2 g fibre)
1 g protein
5 g total fat (0 g saturated fat)
120 mg sodium
75 calories

dinner menu #15

Dilled Carrot Slaw

Dill adds its own unique flavour to this tangy cabbage salad.

4 1/2 cups	shredded cabbage	1.125 L
1 1/2 cups	shredded carrots	375 mL
1/3 cup	cider vinegar	75 mL
1/3 cup	light mayonnaise	75 mL
1/4 tsp	low-calorie sweetener	1 mL
1/4 tsp	dry dillweed	1 mL
1/4 tsp	each: salt and freshly ground pepper	1 mL

1 In large bowl, combine cabbage and carrots. Whisk together vinegar, mayonnaise, sweetener, dillweed, salt and pepper. Toss with cabbage mixture until coated.

Makes 6 servings, 6 cups (1500 mL).

dinner menu #15

Oatmeal and Date Bars

These excellent cookies can go to work, school or dinner for dessert. They are a lower-fat version of matrimonial cake!

3/4 cup	unsweetened applesauce	175 mL
1/2 cup	granular low-calorie sweetener with sucralose	125 mL
1/4 cup	fancy molasses	50 mL
1/4 cup	canola oil	50 mL
1	egg	1
1 tsp	vanilla extract	5 mL
1 1/2 cups	large flake rolled oats	375 mL
1 cup	whole wheat flour	250 mL
1/4 cup	wheat germ	50 mL
1/4 cup	skim milk powder	50 mL
1 tsp	ground cinnamon	5 mL
1/2 tsp	each: baking powder and baking soda	2 mL
1/3 cup	finely chopped dates	75 mL

1 In large bowl, stir together applesauce, sweetener, molasses, oil, egg and vanilla until smooth. Stir in oats, flour, wheat germ, milk powder, cinnamon, baking powder and soda; mix thoroughly. Stir in dates.

2 Spray 13 × 9-inch (3.5 L) baking pan with nonstick vegetable coating; press batter into pan. Bake in 350°F (180°C) oven for 20 minutes or until firm to touch. Cut into 32 bars while still warm.

Makes 32 bars.

PREPARATION TIME:
15 minutes

COOKING TIME:
about 20 minutes

Each serving:
1/16 of recipe, 2 bars

1/2 STARCH CHOICE
1/2 FRUITS & VEGETABLES CHOICE
1/2 SUGARS CHOICE
1 FATS & OILS CHOICE

20 g carbohydrate (2 g fibre)
4 g protein
5 g total fat (1 g saturated fat)
46 mg sodium
129 calories

PREPARATION TIME:
30 minutes

COOKING TIME:
about 1 hour

Each serving:
1 1/3 cups (325 mL)

1/2 STARCH CHOICE
1 FRUITS & VEGETABLES CHOICE
3 PROTEIN CHOICES
1 EXTRA

24 g carbohydrate (5 g fibre)
23 g protein
8 g total fat (2 g saturated fat)
665 mg sodium
251 calories

KITCHEN TIP

The amount of lamb stated is weight after trimming. You'll need to buy extra since there will be some trimming of fat.

To remove excess fat, chill the soup, then reheat before serving.

dinner menu #16
Hearty Lamb Scotch Broth

This is truly "a meal in a bowl." Make it when you simply do not have time to prepare a full meat and vegetable meal. A serving is a high source of fibre, an excellent source of vitamin A, niacin and B12.

1 lb	lean lamb, trimmed and cubed (see Tip)	500 g
1 cup	chopped onion	250 mL
3	cloves garlic, thinly sliced	3
6 cups	sodium-reduced beef broth	1.5 L
1/2 cup	pot barley	125 mL
1/4 cup	finely chopped fresh dill OR 1 tbsp (15 mL) dried	50 mL
2 tbsp	tomato paste	25 mL
2	bay leaves	2
1 tsp	dried thyme leaves	5 mL
1/4 tsp	freshly ground pepper	1 mL
1 cup	sliced carrots	250 mL
1 cup	sliced parsnips	250 mL

1 In large saucepan on medium-high heat, brown lamb, onion and garlic for 10 minutes, stirring often. Remove to large saucepan.

2 Add beef broth, barley, dill, tomato paste, bay leaves, thyme and pepper. Bring to a boil, reduce heat, cover and simmer for 45 minutes. Add carrots and parsnips; cook for 15 minutes or until vegetables and lamb are tender. Discard bay leaves before serving (see Tip).

Makes 6 servings, 8 cups (2 L).

dinner menu #17

Double Cheese 'n Ham Casserole

This make-ahead casserole can be refrigerated until 45 minutes before dinner.

2	egg whites	2
1	egg	1
1 cup	shredded light mozzarella cheese	250 mL
3/4 cup	diced cooked ham	175 mL
2/3 cup	light ricotta cheese	150 mL
1/2 cup	skim milk	125 mL
1/4 cup	all purpose flour	50 mL
2 tbsp	chopped fresh parsley	25 mL
1/2 tsp	hot pepper sauce	2 mL
Pinch	each: salt and freshly ground pepper	Pinch
1 tsp	soft margarine OR butter	5 mL
2/3 cup	sliced mushrooms (3 large)	150 mL
2	green onions, sliced	2
1/4 cup	chopped sweet red pepper	50 mL
	Paprika	

PREPARATION TIME:
20 minutes

COOKING TIME:
about 35 minutes

Each serving:
1/4 of recipe

1/2 STARCH CHOICE
1/2 MILK SKIM CHOICE
1 1/2 PROTEIN CHOICES
1 FATS & OILS CHOICE

12 g carbohydrate (1 g fibre)
24 g protein
12 g total fat (6 g saturated fat)
654 mg sodium
256 calories

1 In medium bowl, beat together egg whites and egg. Stir in mozzarella, ham, ricotta cheese, milk, flour, parsley, hot pepper sauce, salt and pepper.

2 In nonstick skillet, melt margarine over medium-high heat; cook mushrooms, onions and red pepper for 5 minutes or until vegetables are tender.

3 Spray 9-inch (23 cm) pie plate with nonstick vegetable coating. Place vegetables in bottom of pan. Spoon in egg mixture; sprinkle with paprika. Cover and refrigerate until baking time.

4 Bake in 350°F (180°C) oven for 40 minutes or until set and top is golden brown. Let stand for 5 minutes before cutting.

Makes 4 servings.

PREPARATION TIME:
10 minutes

COOKING TIME:
10 minutes

Each serving:
2 slices

1 STARCH CHOICE
1/2 FATS & OILS CHOICE
1 EXTRA

18 g carbohydrate (1 g fibre)
3 g protein
3 g total fat (0 g saturated fat)
175 mg sodium
107 calories

dinner menu #17

Warm Garlic Bread

Italian herbs are the crowning touch to this satisfying garlic bread.

8	slices French bread stick (120 g total)	8
2 tsp	olive oil	10 mL
4	small cloves garlic, minced	4
1/2 tsp	Italian herbs	2 mL

1 Arrange bread slices on a baking pan. Combine oil and garlic. Brush lightly over bread surfaces. Sprinkle with herbs.

2 Bake in 350°F (180°C) oven for 10 minutes or until bread is golden and toasted.

Makes 4 servings, 8 slices.

dinner menu #17

Fast and Healthy Apple Crisp

There is lots of fibre in this crisp from the natural bran in the topping and the unpeeled apples.

4	medium apples, unpeeled	4
1/4 cup	natural bran	50 mL
4 tsp	all purpose flour	20 mL
4 tsp	brown sugar	20 mL
1/2 tsp	vanilla extract	2 mL
Pinch	each: ground nutmeg and cinnamon	Pinch

1 Core and slice apples. Arrange in shallow microwave-safe casserole.

2 In small bowl, combine bran, flour, sugar, vanilla, nutmeg and cinnamon. Sprinkle evenly over apples.

3 Microwave on High (100%) for 5 minutes or until apples are tender OR bake in 350°F (180°C) oven for 35 minutes or until apples bubble up around edge.

Makes 4 servings.

PREPARATION TIME:
10 minutes

COOKING TIME:
about 5 minutes

Each serving:
1/4 of recipe

2 FRUITS & VEGETABLES CHOICES
1/2 SUGARS CHOICE

31 g carbohydrate (5 g fibre)
1 g protein
1 g total fat (0 g saturated fat)
1 mg sodium
126 calories

PREPARATION TIME:
10 minutes

COOKING TIME:
about 3 minutes on each side

Each serving:
1/4 of recipe

3 PROTEIN CHOICES

0 g carbohydrate
21 g protein
8 g total fat (2 g saturated fat)
89 mg sodium
162 calories

dinner menu #18

Asian Grilled Pork Tenderloin

Combine the leanest and most tender of all pork cuts with Asian flavourings for a fast and enjoyable meal.

4 tsp	sesame oil	20 mL
8	slices pork tenderloin (400 g raw)	8
1 tbsp	lime juice	15 mL
1 tsp	sodium-reduced soy sauce	5 mL
	Freshly ground pepper	
	Chopped fresh cilantro (Chinese parsley)	

1 In nonstick skillet, heat oil on medium-high heat; cook pork for 3 minutes, turn and cook for 3 minutes or until pork is browned. Drizzle with lime juice and soy sauce. Sprinkle with pepper and cilantro and serve.

Makes 4 servings.

dinner menu #18

Vegetable Kebabs

Cooking vegetables on skewers ensures their quick and even cooking.

12	zucchini cubes	12
8	cherry tomatoes	8
16	whole mushrooms	16
1/4 cup	calorie-reduced Italian salad dressing	50 mL

1 Place zucchini, tomatoes and mushrooms in a plastic bag. Drizzle with salad dressing. Close bag and shake to coat vegetables.

2 Remove vegetables from bag and, alternating vegetables, thread on skewers. Broil or grill for 5 minutes or until vegetables are cooked.

Makes 4 servings.

PREPARATION TIME:
10 minutes

COOKING TIME:
about 5 minutes

Each serving:
1 skewer

1/2 FRUITS & VEGETABLES CHOICE

6 g carbohydrate (2 g fibre)
2 g protein
1 g total fat (0 g saturated fat)
218 mg sodium
35 calories

PREPARATION TIME:
10 minutes

COOKING TIME:
about 6 minutes

Each serving:
1/4 of recipe

1/2 STARCH CHOICE
3 PROTEIN CHOICES

9 g carbohydrate (1 g fibre)
22 g protein
9 g total fat (4 g saturated fat)
146 mg sodium
237 calories

dinner menu #20

Calves' Liver with Onion and Herbs

All liver lovers will adore this old favourite, liver with herbs and onions. It can be on the table in under 15 minutes.

4 tsp	canola oil	20 mL
2	small onions, chopped	2
4	pieces calves' liver (each 120 g raw)	4
2 1/2 tbsp	all purpose flour	32 mL
1/4 tsp	ground thyme	1 mL
	Salt and freshly ground pepper	

1 In nonstick skillet, heat oil on medium-high heat; cook onions for 2 minutes or until golden. Remove from skillet; keep warm.

2 Shake liver in flour, thyme, salt and pepper. Cook in skillet for 2 minutes per side or just until cooked and golden.

3 Top liver with onions and serve.

Makes 4 servings.

dinner menu #21

Spanish Omelette

Filled with onions, tomatoes and mushrooms, this classic **Spanish Omelette** is a quick and easy dinner.

1	green onion, sliced	1
1/2	small tomato, chopped	1/2
2	medium mushrooms, sliced	2
1/2 tsp	soft margarine OR butter	2 mL
2	eggs	2
2 tbsp	water	25 mL

1 In nonstick skillet, melt margarine on medium-high; sauté onion, tomato and mushrooms for 5 minutes or until vegetables are cooked. Set aside.

2 Beat eggs and water together. Add to skillet and cook until eggs are set. Fill omelette with vegetable mixture and serve.

Makes 1 serving.

PREPARATION TIME:
10 minutes

COOKING TIME:
about 8 minutes

Each serving:
1 omelette

1/2 FRUITS & VEGETABLES CHOICE
2 PROTEIN CHOICES
1 FATS & OILS CHOICE

6 g carbohydrate (1 g fibre)
14 g protein
12 g total fat (3 g saturated fat)
160 mg sodium
189 calories

PREPARATION TIME:
20 minutes

COOKING TIME:
15 minutes

Each serving:
1/2 of recipe (1/2 chicken fingers
and 1/3 cup/75 mL dip)

2 1/2 STARCH CHOICES
3 PROTEIN CHOICES

39 g carbohydrate (1 g fibre)
27 g protein
4 g total fat (1 g saturated fat)
1067 mg sodium
308 calories

1 Cut chicken breasts lengthwise into 1-inch (2.5 cm) strips.

2 In shallow dish, combine 1/4 cup (50 mL) undiluted soup and 2 tbsp (25 mL) milk.

3 In plastic bag, combine cornflake crumbs, dill and pepper. Dip chicken pieces into soup mixture, then into crumbs.

4 Spray baking pan with nonstick vegetable coating. Arrange chicken pieces separately on pan.

5 Bake in 375°F (190°C) oven for about 15 minutes or until chicken is crisp and no longer pink inside.

dinner menu #22

Crispy Chicken Fingers with Creamy Dipping Sauce

Crisped fingers of low-fat chicken breast dipped in a dreamy creamy sauce make a delicious fast-start to a healthy dinner.

2	boneless skinless chicken breast halves (200 g raw)	2
1/2	can (284 mL) half fat cream of mushroom soup, divided	1/2
1/4 cup	low-fat milk, divided	50 mL
3/4 cup	corn flake crumbs	175 mL
2 tsp	dried dill OR 2 tbsp (25 mL) chopped fresh dill	10 mL
1/8 tsp	freshly ground pepper	0.5 mL
1 tbsp	ketchup	15 mL
1/4 tsp	Worcestershire sauce	1 mL

6 **Creamy Dipping Sauce:** Whisk together remaining soup, milk, ketchup and Worcestershire sauce. Microwave on Medium (70%) until mixture is warm. Divide sauce into two small bowls to dip chicken fingers.

Makes 2 servings and about 2/3 cup (150 mL) sauce.

dinner menu #22

Baked Sliced Apples

Apples are a great dessert choice. Their mellow goodness is cooked with cinnamon and sour cream in this recipe.

2 cups	sliced unpeeled apples (2 medium)	500 mL
1/4 cup	granulated brown low-calorie sweetener	50 mL
2 tsp	soft margarine OR butter	10 mL
1 tsp	vanilla extract	5 mL
1/4 tsp	ground cinnamon	1 mL
1/4 cup	low-fat sour cream	50 mL

1   Place apples in shallow microwave-safe casserole. Sprinkle with sweetener. Add margarine, vanilla and cinnamon.

2   Cover loosely with plastic wrap. Microwave at Medium (70 %) for 5 minutes or until apples are tender. Spoon sour cream around edges; cook for 1 minute. Serve warm.

Makes 2 servings.

PREPARATION TIME:
10 minutes

COOKING TIME:
about 6 minutes

Each serving:
1/2 of recipe

2 FRUITS & VEGETABLES CHOICES
1 FATS & OILS CHOICE

21 g carbohydrate (2 g fibre)
2 g protein
6 g total fat (1 g saturated fat)
61 mg sodium
132 calories

APPLE TIPS

A medium apple has about 80 calories and is a good source of vitamin A, fibre (providing you eat the skin) and potassium. Over 80% of the fibre in apples is soluble fibre in the form of pectin. Studies have shown that pectin and other soluble fibres lower cholesterol levels and slow the digestion of carbohydrate into glucose sugar.

Cortland, Spy and Ida Red varieties are excellent all-purpose apples.

PREPARATION TIME:
10 minutes

COOKING TIME:
20 minutes

Each serving:
2 eggs with topping and one English muffin

**1 1/2 STARCH CHOICES
1/2 FRUITS & VEGETABLES
CHOICE
3 PROTEIN CHOICES
1 FATS & OILS CHOICE**

32 g carbohydrate (5 g fibre)
23 g protein
14 g total fat (5 g saturated fat)
599 mg sodium
336 calories

For Single Serving

Break two eggs into medium custard cup sprayed with nonstick vegetable coating. Top with 1/2 of tomato and milk mixture and cheese as directed in recipe. Place custard cup on small baking pan and bake as directed.

dinner menu #23
Baked Eggs with Tomato

Eggs are not only for breakfast! Oven-poached in milk with a basil-tomato topping and a cheese garnish, they are just right for an easy-to-make light dinner. Properly stored, eggs will keep four to five weeks.

4	eggs	4
3/4 cup	diced tomato (about 1 medium)	175 mL
2 tsp	chopped fresh basil OR 1 tsp (5 mL) dried	10 mL
2 tbsp	low-fat milk	25 mL
1/8 tsp	freshly ground pepper	0.5 mL
1/4 cup	shredded light old Cheddar cheese	50 mL
2	whole wheat English muffins, split and toasted	2

1 Spray shallow casserole with nonstick vegetable coating. Break eggs, one at a time, into casserole. Combine tomato and basil. Top each egg with some of the tomato mixture.

2 Combine milk and pepper; pour over tomato mixture. Sprinkle eggs evenly with cheese.

3 Bake in 350°F (180°C) oven for 20 minutes or until eggs are set. Serve each egg on 1/2 toasted English muffin.

Makes 2 servings.

dinner menu #24

Oven Beef Stew with Vegetables

Beef stew is best made in larger amounts. Flavours are better and several meals are ready from the one effort. Freeze the leftovers or invite friends over for a hearty winter meal. Lean beef fits well into a lower-fat diet. And this recipe keeps lean beef lean by using low-fat cooking methods.

1/4 cup	all purpose flour	50 mL
1/2 tsp	each: celery seed and paprika	2 mL
1/4 tsp	freshly ground pepper	1 mL
1 1/4 lb	lean stewing beef	625 g
1 tbsp	canola oil	15 mL
1 1/4 cups	water	300 mL
1	pkg (36 g) onion soup mix	1
1 tbsp	horseradish	15 mL
3	small onions, cut in half	3
1 cup	rutabaga OR carrot chunks (1/2-inch/1 cm thick)	250 mL
2 cups	small whole button mushrooms	500 mL

PREPARATION TIME:
20 minutes

COOKING TIME:
about 2 hours

Each serving:
1 cup (250 mL)

1 1/2 FRUITS & VEGETABLES CHOICES
2 1/2 PROTEIN CHOICES

16 g carbohydrate (3 g fibre)
20 g protein
6 g total fat (1 g saturated fat)
577 mg sodium
198 calories

1 Combine flour, celery seed, paprika and pepper in plastic bag. Trim and discard all visible fat from beef. Cut into even-size cubes. Lightly toss beef in seasoned flour; reserve excess flour.

2 Add oil to 8 cup (2 L) oven-proof casserole. Place casserole in 450°F (230°C) oven for 5 minutes. Remove casserole; add beef, separating cubes. Return to oven and brown meat, uncovered, for 15 minutes; stir once.

3 Remove casserole from oven. Reduce oven temperature to 350°F (180°C). Combine water, soup mix, horseradish and reserved flour; pour over meat. Return casserole to oven; cover and bake for 1 hour, stirring once. Add onions, rutabaga, mushrooms and extra water, if needed. Bake, covered, for 45 minutes or until meat and vegetables are tender.

Makes about 6 servings, 6 cups (1.5 L).

PREPARATION TIME:
15 minutes

COOKING TIME:
about 35 minutes

Each serving:
about 1 cup (50 mL)

2 STARCH CHOICES
1 FATS & OILS CHOICE

36 g carbohydrate (4 g fibre)
4 g protein
5 g total fat (1 g saturated fat)
184 mg sodium
196 calories

dinner menu #25

Scalloped Sweet and White Potatoes

Sweet potatoes are added to white potatoes for a dynamite variation. Both potato varieties are a source of fibre and full of great nutrients. We use broth instead of milk for fewer calories and more flavour.

1 cup	thinly sliced white potatoes (2 small)	250 mL
1 cup	thinly sliced sweet potatoes (1/2 small)	250 mL
1/2	small onion, thinly sliced, divided	1/2
	Freshly ground pepper	
1/3 cup	chicken OR vegetable broth	75 mL
2 tsp	soft margarine OR butter	10 mL
1/4 tsp	ground nutmeg	1 mL

1 Lightly spray two small baking pans or casseroles with nonstick vegetable coating.

2 In medium bowl, combine white and sweet potato slices. Place one-quarter of the potatoes in each prepared pan. Top with one-quarter of onion and sprinkle lightly with pepper. Repeat layers.

3 Heat broth and margarine to boiling; pour over potatoes. Sprinkle with nutmeg.

4 Cover each pan with foil. Bake in 350°F (180°C) oven for 25 minutes. Uncover and bake for 15 minutes or until tender and golden brown.

Makes 2 servings, about 2 cups (500 mL).

dinner menu #25

Pineapple Smoothie Dessert

Instant pudding mix allows a busy cook to have this attractive and tasty dessert ready in just 10 minutes.

1	pkg (30 g) vanilla light instant pudding mix with aspartame	1
1 cup	unsweetened canned crushed pineapple in juice	250 mL
1 cup	low-fat (1%) plain yogurt	250 mL
4	large strawberries for garnish (see Tip)	4

1 In medium bowl, combine pudding mix and pineapple with juice. Beat with wire whisk for 2 minutes. Stir in yogurt. Divide evenly between 4 serving dishes. Garnish with strawberries.

Makes 4 servings, 2 cups (500 mL).

PREPARATION TIME:
10 minutes

Each serving:
1/2 cup (125 mL)

1/2 STARCH CHOICE
1 FRUITS & VEGETABLES CHOICE
1/2 MILK 1% CHOICE

20 g carbohydrate (1 g fibre)
4 g protein
0 g total fat
367 mg sodium
93 calories

KITCHEN TIP

Frozen unsweetened strawberries can be substituted for fresh.

PREPARATION TIME:
10 minutes

COOKING TIME:
about 10 minutes

Each serving:
1 cup (250 mL)

1 STARCH CHOICE
3 1/2 PROTEIN CHOICES

18 g carbohydrate (3 g fibre)
26 g protein
8 g total fat (1 g saturated fat)
1539 mg sodium, 263 calories

Tuna Variation

Replace expensive crabmeat with 1/2 can (170 g) drained water-packed tuna. Use remaining tuna in a sandwich.

Makes 2 servings, about 2 cups (500 mL).

Each serving:
1 cup (250 mL

1 STARCH CHOICE
3 1/2 PROTEIN CHOICES

18 g carbohydrate (3 g fibre)
26 g protein
7 g total fat (0 g saturated fat)
1151 mg sodium, 260 calories

KITCHEN TIPS

Use about 2/3 cup (150 mL) frozen shrimp to replace canned shrimp.

Chopped fresh parsley enhances the flavour of almost any savoury dish.

dinner menu #26
Mushroom Seafood Strogonoff

Just combine two cans of seafood, a can of creamy mushroom soup, some mushrooms and green peas to create this elegant version of a traditional Stroganoff. It's an easy-to-prepare dinner to proudly serve to company.

1	can (10 oz/284 mL) half-fat cream of mushroom condensed soup	1
1	can (120 g) crabmeat, drained	1
1	can (106 g) shrimp, drained (see Tip)	1
1 tsp	canola oil	5 mL
1 1/2 cups	sliced mushrooms	375 mL
1/2 cup	frozen peas	125 mL
2 tbsp	sherry, optional	25 mL
	Chopped fresh parsley (see Tip)	

1 In medium saucepan, combine undiluted soup, crabmeat and shrimp; set aside.

2 In nonstick skillet, heat oil on medium-high. Add mushrooms and sauté for 5 minutes or until brown.

3 Stir mushrooms into seafood mixture; heat over medium-low until mixture is hot. Stir in peas and sherry, if using and continue to heat until peas are thawed and cooked, stirring frequently.

Makes 2 servings, about 2 cups (500 mL) seafood.

dinner menu #27

Veal Cutlets in Tomato Herb Sauce

Cooking veal in a sauce and by moist heat keeps this lower-fat meat juicy.

1	veal cutlet (200 g)	1
1 tsp	olive oil	5 mL
1/2 cup	sliced mushrooms	125 mL
1/2 cup	canned tomato sauce	125 mL
1/4 tsp	each: dried basil and oregano	1 mL

1 Heat oil in nonstick skillet on medium-high. Sauté meat until golden on both sides, being careful not to overcook. Remove and reserve.

2 Add mushrooms to skillet; sauté for 5 minutes or until golden brown. Return meat to skillet, spoon mushrooms over meat, top with tomato sauce, basil and oregano. Reduce heat to medium-low, cover and cook for 5 minutes or until meat is cooked and sauce hot. Cut meat into 2 servings and spoon sauce and mushrooms over each.

Makes 2 servings.

PREPARATION TIME:
5 minutes

COOKING TIME:
about 10 minutes

Each serving:
1/2 of recipe

1/2 FRUITS & VEGETABLES CHOICE
3 1/2 PROTEIN CHOICES

3 g carbohydrate (1 g fibre)
23 g protein
5 g total fat (2 g saturated fat)
198 mg sodium
150 calories

PREPARATION TIME:
5 minutes

COOKING TIME:
about 10 minutes

Each serving:
1 fillet

3 PROTEIN CHOICES

1 g carbohydrate (0 g fibre)
19 g protein
6 g total fat (0 g saturated fat)
51 mg sodium
135 calories

K I T C H E N   T I P

The microwave oven also cooks fish very well due to the high moisture content of fish. This amount of fish will require about 5 minutes cooking on High (100%) power.

dinner menu #28

Baked Whitefish

This simple recipe lets the fresh flavours of the fish predominate. Be sure to use the freshest fish available for best results. Turbot, sole or rainbow trout can be substituted for whitefish.

2	fillets whitefish (200 g raw)	2
2 tsp	lemon juice	10 mL
Pinch	dried thyme	Pinch
	Salt and freshly ground pepper	

1 Place fillets on a baking pan sprayed with non-stick vegetable coating. Drizzle with lemon juice and sprinkle lightly with thyme, salt and pepper.

2 Bake in 400°F (200°C) oven for 10 minutes per inch (2.5 cm) thickness or until fish is opaque.

Makes 2 servings.

dinner menu #28

Rosemary Roasted Potatoes

Crisp on the outside, full of garlic and rosemary flavours and fragrances, potatoes just don't come any better! But it's important to choose the right potato variety. Yukon Gold potatoes are a good choice.

2	unpeeled medium (95 g each) potatoes, halved	2
1–2	cloves garlic, minced	1–2
1 tbsp	olive oil	15 mL
1 tbsp	chopped fresh rosemary OR 1/2 tsp (2 mL) dried	15 mL

1 Toss potatoes in mixture of garlic, oil and rosemary, being careful to press solids onto surface. Place on baking pan and roast in 400°F (200°C) oven for 30 minutes or until potatoes are tender.

Makes 2 servings.

PREPARATION TIME:
5 minutes

COOKING TIME:
30 minutes

Each serving:
1/2 of recipe

1 STARCH CHOICE
1 1/2 FATS & OILS CHOICES

17 g carbohydrate (2 g fibre)
2 g protein
7 g total fat (1 g saturated fat)
7 mg sodium
135 calories

GARLIC TIPS

Store garlic bulbs in a cool, dry, well-ventilated place. Avoid storing in the refrigerator as garlic odour could spread to other foods.

Choose bulbs that are firm, plump, non-sprouted and unshrivelled. The papery skin around each clove should be completely closed.

Light Lemon Mousse

Tangy fresh lemon makes this a very refreshing dessert. It reminds us of the Lemon Snow of our childhood.

1	lemon	1
1/4 cup	granular low-calorie sweetener with sucralose	50 mL
2	eggs, separated	2
1/2 cup	water	125 mL
1 tsp	unflavoured gelatin	5 mL
1 tbsp	granulated sugar	15 mL

PREPARATION TIME:
about 35 minutes

CHILL:
30 minutes

Each serving:
1/2 cup (125 mL)

1/2 SUGARS CHOICE
1/2 PROTEIN CHOICE
1 EXTRA

7 g carbohydrate (0 g fibre)
4 g protein
3 g total fat (1 g saturated fat)
34 mg sodium
66 calories

Variation: Light Orange Mousse

For a flavour change, replace lemon with the same amount of orange rind and juice.

1 Grate rind from lemon and reserve. Squeeze lemon; measure 1/4 cup (50 mL) juice.

2 In small microwave-safe bowl, combine rind, juice, sweetener, egg yolks and water. Sprinkle gelatin over top and stir into mixture; let stand for 1 minute to soften.

3 Microwave at Medium (70%) for 4 minutes or until mixture is slightly thickened and gelatin is dissolved; stir frequently.

4 Transfer to metal bowl and freeze for 30 minutes or until mixture becomes thickened; stir several times.

5 Beat egg whites with sugar until stiff peaks form. Fold into lemon mixture and pour into 4 dessert dishes. Chill before serving.

Makes 4 servings, 2 cups (500 mL).

dinner menu #29

Herbed Chicken and Vegetables

Onions, garlic, rosemary and marjoram pep up this colourful stovetop stew. Chock full of healthy vegetables, it is another great use of low-fat skinless chicken breasts. Add extra liquid if too thick.

1 tbsp	canola oil	15 mL
1	small onion, chopped	1
1	clove garlic, minced	1
2	small (200 g) boneless, skinless chicken breast halves, cubed	2
1/2 tsp	each: dried rosemary and marjoram	2 mL
1/8 tsp	each: salt and freshly ground pepper	0.5 mL
1/4 cup	chicken broth	50 mL
1 cup	canned crushed tomatoes	250 mL
1 cup	cubed squash (see Tip)	250 mL
1/2	sweet green pepper, coarsely chopped	1/2
1 cup	halved button mushrooms	250 mL

1 In large nonstick skillet, heat oil over medium-high. Add onion and garlic; cook for 5 minutes or until softened.

2 Add chicken to skillet. Sauté for 3 minutes or until lightly browned. Sprinkle with rosemary, marjoram, salt and pepper. Stir in broth, tomatoes, squash, green pepper and mushrooms. Bring to boil, cover, reduce heat to low and cook for about 20 minutes or until squash is tender.

Makes 2 servings, 2 1/4 cups (550 mL).

PREPARATION TIME:
15 minutes

COOKING TIME:
about 25 minutes

Each serving:
about 1 cup (250 mL)

1 1/2 FRUITS & VEGETABLES CHOICES
3 PROTEIN CHOICES

19 g carbohydrate (**4 g fibre**)
20 g protein
9 g total fat (1 g saturated fat)
608 mg sodium
223 calories

KITCHEN TIP

Butternut squash is ideal for this recipe. It's available in the produce section of your supermarket, whole or cut up in smaller amounts.

PREPARATION TIME:
10 minutes

Each serving:
1 tbsp (15 mL) dressing

1 FATS & OILS CHOICE

1 g carbohydrate (0 g fibre)
0 g protein
5 g total fat (1 g saturated fat)
58 mg sodium
49 calories

DRESSING TIPS

Today we are able to buy sherry vinegar quite readily. However, red wine or cider vinegar can substitute for sherry, but the resulting flavour will be quite different.

Refrigerate the dressing to use on several salads.

Using olive oil adds monounsaturated fat to your diet (a good thing to do).

dinner menu #29

Warm Sherry Vinaigrette

Sherry vinegar is a fast-growing addition to the specialty vinegar family. Good ones are not cheap, but a little goes a long way. This Spanish import tastes nutty and mellow compared to its more piquant cousins. Fresh spinach, so high in vitamin A and so low in calories, makes an excellent salad green to toss with the dressing.

1/4 cup	extra virgin olive oil	50 mL
1/4 cup	sherry vinegar (see Tip)	50 mL
3 tbsp	water	45 mL
1	green onion, thinly sliced	1
1/4 tsp	each: salt and sweetener	1 mL
1/8 tsp	freshly ground pepper	0.5 mL

1 In container with tight-fitting lid, combine oil, vinegar, water, onion, salt, sweetener and pepper; shake well and refrigerate.

2 Warm in microwave on Medium (70%) for about 30 seconds just before tossing with the salad greens.

Makes about 2/3 cup (150 mL) dressing.

dinner menu #29

Raspberry Cream Dessert

When raspberries are in season, we just can't eat enough of these succulent summer delicacies.

1 cup	whole raspberries (see Tip)	250 mL
2 tsp	unflavoured gelatin	10 mL
1/2 cup	low-fat milk	125 mL
2/3 cup	low-fat French vanilla yogurt sweetened with aspartame OR sucralose (see Tip)	150 mL
2 tsp	granulated sugar	10 mL
	Whole raspberries	

1 In blender or food processor, purée raspberries until almost smooth; remove and set aside.

2 Sprinkle gelatin over milk in small saucepan or microwave-safe dish. Heat until gelatin is completely dissolved. Stir into puréed fruit; add yogurt and sugar and stir to blend. Pour into 3 dessert dishes; refrigerate, for about 1 hour, or until set. (See Tip.)

3 Garnish with extra whole raspberries.

Makes 3 servings, 1 3/4 cups (425 mL).

PREPARATION TIME:
10 minutes

CHILL:
about 1 hour

Each serving:
1/3 of recipe

1/2 FRUITS & VEGETABLES CHOICE
1 MILK 1% CHOICE

14 g carbohydrate (2 g fibre)
5 g protein
1 g total fat (0 g saturated fat)
46 mg sodium
78 calories

KITCHEN TIPS

For faster chilling, set dishes in freezer section of refrigerator.

You can replace commercial low-fat French vanilla yogurt with 2/3 cup (150 mL) of our **Homemade Vanilla Yogurt** (page 53).

RASPBERRY TIP

Raspberries are very fragile and should be used within a day or two of purchase.

PREPARATION TIME:
20 minutes

COOKING TIME:
about 1 1/2 hours

Each serving:
2 to 3 slices (60 g) cooked turkey
and 1/2 cup (125 mL) stuffing

**1/2 STARCH CHOICE
3 PROTEIN CHOICES
1 EXTRA**

11 g carbohydrate (1 g fibre)
21 g protein
7 g total fat (1 g saturated fat)
328 mg sodium
188 calories

TURKEY TIP

Before roasting, pull skin back from breast and remove as much visible fat as possible. Then pull skin back over meat to keep meat moist while roasting.

1 In a nonstick skillet, on medium-high, sauté onion, celery and mushrooms in margarine for 5 minutes or until softened. Remove from heat and stir in apple, seasonings, breadcrumbs and pecans. Set aside.

2 Clean and prepare turkey breast for stuffing.

dinner menu #30
Roast Turkey Breast with Stuffing

Make an old-fashioned meal of roast turkey with stuffing, but without all the trouble of doing a whole bird. And with less leftover turkey! Leave the skin on during cooking for maximum taste and tenderness.

2 1/2 lb	whole turkey breast (see Tip)	1.5 kg
Stuffing		
1/2 cup	each: chopped onion and celery	125 mL
6	small mushrooms, chopped	6
1 tbsp	soft margarine OR butter	15 mL
1/2 cup	chopped apple	125 mL
1/2 tsp	each: dried thyme leaves and salt	2 mL
1/4 tsp	freshly ground pepper	1 mL
2 cups	breadcrumbs (day old)	500 mL
2 tbsp	chopped pecans	25 mL

3 Fill turkey cavity with stuffing; turn over onto a piece of aluminum foil large enough to draw edges up around the turkey breast. Punch holes in foil to allow any fat to drain. Place turkey on rack in shallow roasting pan.

4 Roast in 350°F (180°C) oven for 45 minutes. Pull foil away from meat to allow browning. Roast for 45 minutes longer or until meat thermometer registers 170°F (75°C) in thickest part.

5 Remove from oven; let stand loosely covered with foil for 10 minutes before carving. Remove skin and discard. Serve stuffing and sliced meat on warm serving plates.

Makes 3 cups (750 mL) stuffing and enough turkey to serve 6 to 8.

dinner menu #30

Light Cranberry Sauce

Although cranberry is the traditional sauce for chicken or turkey, it goes equally well with other meats and casseroles. This very fast and easy-to-prepare "light" version is made without sugar.

2 cups	cranberries, fresh or frozen (see Tip)	250 mL
1/2 cup	water	125 mL
1 tsp	shredded orange rind	5 mL
3–4 tbsp	low-calorie sweetener	45–60 mL

1 Place cranberries, water and orange rind in 2 cup (500 mL) glass measure. Cover loosely with plastic wrap. Microwave on High (100%) for 3 minutes; stir. Microwave on Medium (70%) for 2 minutes or until thickened; cool slightly.

2 Stir in sweetener to taste. Cover and refrigerate for up to 1 week.

Makes about 1 cup (250 mL).

PREPARATION TIME:
5 minutes

COOKING TIME:
about 5 minutes

Each serving:
2 tbsp (25 mL)

1/2 FRUITS & VEGETABLES CHOICE

4 g carbohydrate (1 g fibre)
0 g protein
0 g total fat
1 mg sodium
16 calories

KITCHEN TIP

Fresh cranberries store well—one month in the refrigerator and one year in the freezer. Freeze them unwashed in their bags. Wash just the amount you need before using.

snacks

Why do we snack? Because we're hungry, bored, anxious or just need an energy boost? But if you have diabetes, there's an even better reason. Studies have shown that spreading the food you need over several small meals a day improves diabetes control by smoothing out blood glucose highs and lows. And, if you need to lose some weight, a snack can keep you satisfied between meals and discourage overeating at the next meal.

How much **should you snack?** To begin with, eating breakfast, lunch and dinner from any of our menus gives you about 1200 calories of food energy per day. This is a significant weight loss path for most people, and you may need more calories. How much more? Your dietitian will recommend an energy intake based on your age, activity level and weight goal (see "How to Use This Book," page 11). You then plan whatever snacks are required to make up any difference between the basic 1200 calories and your prescribed calorie intake. Our snacks come in small (75-calorie), medium (150-calorie) and large (300-calorie) sizes so you can choose just what you need.

When **should you snack?** Planning a snack when you have a long stretch between meals, usually four hours or more, keeps your appetite under control as well as ensuring that your blood glucose doesn't dip uncomfortably low. This means planning to have mid-morning, mid-afternoon or bedtime snacks within the total calories allowed by your meal plan. Those taking insulin or pills for their diabetes may find that a mid-afternoon snack or a bedtime snack helps protect against hypoglycemia (low blood sugar) (see Appendix 1, page 224). Doing a blood glucose test can help you decide.

Our snacks are suitable for the usual snacking times. You'll find snacks to go with tea or coffee (**Date 'n Raisin Soft Cookies** on page 186) or to bring from home (**Popcorn Munch** on page 180). A delayed meal, perhaps on a social occasion, is another time for planning to have one of our before-meal appetizers (**Curried Cheddar Spread** on page 182).

What **foods make good snack choices?** Good choices should be part of a healthy lifestyle. Did you know that a large bag of potato chips usually contains 6 tbsp (90 mL) or 80 grams of fat? That's more than anyone should get from all the food they eat in a whole day. Pretzels, air-popped corn, **Snack Scramble** (page 188) or **Pita Cheese Crisps** (page 181) are all lower fat choices with few calories.

Healthy snacks are a great way to get more complex carbohydrate and fibre in your diet. But that's not all! Whole grain products such as low-fat whole wheat crackers and cereals provide B vitamins as well. Try our **Double Bran Muffins** (page 46) or **Cranberry Scones** (page 191) made with whole wheat flour, or the **Carrot Raisin Oat Cookies** (page190) made with rolled oats. **Hummus Dip with Tortilla Snackers** (page 187) is a high-fibre vegetarian dip with a low glycemic index (see page 4).

Many vegetables and fruits provide beta carotene (vitamin A) and vitamin C as well as fibre and minerals. Our **Garden Tomato Salsa** (page 192) will wake up your taste buds!

Low-fat protein foods and dairy products add satisfaction to a complex carbohydrate snack and help it digest more slowly and last longer—important when you choose a bedtime snack.

snack menus

Snack menus provide either:

> 75 calories (with 10–15 g carbohydrate)
>
> OR 150 calories (with 15–20 g carbohydrate)
>
> OR 300 calories (with 35–40 g carbohydrate)

75-Calorie Snack Menus

menu #1
1/2 cup (125 mL) O-shaped oat cereal
1/4 cup (50 mL) low-fat milk

menu #2
4 tortilla chips (12 g)
1/4 cup (50 mL) salsa

menu #3
1/2 orange, sliced
1/4 cup (50 mL) low-fat cottage cheese

menu #4
2 ginger cookies
tea or coffee with milk

menu #5
2/3 cup (150 mL) cubed cantaloupe
1/4 cup (50 mL) vanilla yogurt with aspartame

menu #6
1 large peach
1/4 cup (50 mL) low-fat cottage cheese

menu #7
3/4 cup (175 mL) low-fat flavoured yogurt with aspartame

menu #8
16 thin pretzel sticks
diet soft drink

menu #9
1 digestive cookie
tea or coffee with milk

menu #10   2 tbsp (25 mL) **Salsa Cheese Spread** (page 178)
3 round melba toasts
diet soft drink

menu #11   1/2 cup (125 mL) **Frozen Melon Smoothie** (page 179)

menu #12   1/2 cup (125 mL) **Popcorn Munch** (page 180)
diet soft drink OR
Chilled Lemonade
*juice of 1/2 lemon, 3/4 cup (175 mL) water,
sweetener to taste, ice cubes*

menu #13   3 **Pita Cheese Crisps** (page181)
diet soft drink

menu #14   4 whole wheat soda crackers
tea or coffee with milk

menu #15   1 1/2 cups (375 mL) light microwave popcorn
1 cup (250 mL) low-fat milk

menu #16   1 tbsp (15 mL) **Curried Cheddar Spread** (page 182)
3 whole wheat soda crackers

150-Calorie Snack Menus

menu #1
3 stoned wheat crackers
2 tbsp (25 mL) light cheese spread
tea or coffee with milk

menu #2
1 shredded wheat biscuit
1/2 cup (125 mL) low-fat milk

menu #3
1 cup (250 mL) strawberries
1/4 cup (50 mL) low-fat cottage cheese
4 melba toasts

menu #4
3 graham wafers
1 serving light hot chocolate
follow package directions

menu #5
2 digestive cookies
1/2 cup (125 mL) low-fat milk

menu #6
3 cups (750 mL) light microwave popcorn
1 cup (250 mL) low-fat milk

menu #7
Cinnamon Toast
Combine 1 tsp (5 mL) soft margarine OR *butter, ground cinnamon and sweetener; spread on 1 slice toast*
1/2 cup (125 mL) low-fat milk

menu #8
1 plain waffle, toasted
1/4 cup (50 mL) low-fat cottage cheese
5 sliced strawberries

m e n u # 9   1/2 English muffin (30 g), toasted,
1 tbsp (15 mL) light peanut butter

m e n u # 1 0   2/3 cup (150 mL) cubed cantaloupe OR honeydew
melon
1/2 cup (125 mL) low-fat cottage cheese

m e n u # 1 1   1 medium apple OR pear
1 cube (25 g) Cheddar cheese

m e n u # 1 2   1 slice whole wheat toast
1 tsp (5 mL) soft margarine OR butter
1 serving light hot chocolate
follow package directions

m e n u # 1 3   1 cup (250 mL) chicken noodle soup
6 whole wheat soda crackers

m e n u # 1 4   1 **Buttermilk Scone** (page 183)
1/2 tsp (2 mL) soft margarine OR butter
1 tsp (5 mL) no-sugar-added fruit spread (page 19)
tea or coffee with milk

m e n u # 1 5   1/4 cup (50 mL) **Light Herb Cheese Spread** (page 184)
6 melba toasts

m e n u # 1 6   1 **Multimix Tea Biscuit** (page 185)
1 tsp (5 mL) soft margarine OR butter
2 tbsp (25 mL) no-sugar-added fruit spread (page 19)

m e n u # 1 7   1 oat bran waffle
3 tbsp (45 mL) **Maple Yogurt Sauce** (page 35)

menu #18
1 square (1/12) **Homestyle Gingerbread** (page 121)
1/4 cup (50 mL) low-fat plain yogurt, sweetener to taste,
ground ginger and vanilla extract, if desired

menu #19
1 cup (250 mL) **Frozen Melon Smoothie** (page 179)

menu #20
1/4 cup (50 mL) **Salsa Cheese Spread** (page 178)
6 round snack crackers (20 g)

menu #21
2 **Date 'n Raisin Soft Cookies** (page 186)
OR 2 digestive cookies
1/2 cup (125 mL) low-fat milk

menu #22
1/3 cup (75 mL) **Hummus Dip**
with 6 **Tortilla Snackers** (page 187)

menu #23
1 **Double Bran Muffin** (page 46)
tea or coffee with milk

menu #24
2 tbsp (25 mL) **Curried Cheddar Spread** (page 182)
6 whole wheat soda crackers

menu #25
1 **Raisin Bran Buttermilk Muffin** (page 49)
tea or coffee with milk

menu #26
1/2 cup (125 mL) **Snack Scramble** (page 188)
1/2 cup (125 mL) low-fat milk

menu #27
1 **Banana Muffin** (page 37)
1/2 tsp (2 mL) soft margarine OR butter
tea or coffee with milk

menu #28   1 cup (250 mL) **Popcorn Munch** (page 180)
diet soft drink

menu #29   4 **Bagel Thins** (page189)
1/2 cup (125 mL) low-fat milk

menu #30   2 **Carrot Raisin Oat Cookies** (page 190)
1/2 cup (125 mL) low-fat milk

menu #31   1 **Cranberry Scone** (page 191), warmed
tea or coffee with milk

menu #32   1/2 cup (125 mL) **Garden Tomato Salsa** (page 192)
13 tortilla chips
chilled soda water with lime slice

menu #33   4 **Pita Cheese Crisps** (page 181)
2 celery sticks filled with
2 tbsp (25 mL) light ricotta cheese

300-Calorie Snack Menus

m e n u # 1
1 medium apple OR pear
1/4 cup (50 mL) dry roasted peanuts

m e n u # 2
Homemade Ice Cream Sandwich
2 oatmeal cookies and 1/4 cup (50 mL) light ice cream
1 cup (250 mL) low-fat milk

m e n u # 3
1/2 can tomato soup with water
8 whole wheat soda crackers
3 tbsp (45 mL) light cheese spread

m e n u # 4
1 English muffin OR hot cross bun, toasted
1 tbsp (15 mL) peanut butter
1/2 cup (125 mL) low-fat milk

m e n u # 5
Deli Sandwich
Spread 2 large slices (35 g each) pumpernickel rye bread with 2 tsp (10 mL) soft margarine OR butter; add 1 slice (30 g) turkey or Black Forest ham, mustard and lettuce

m e n u # 6
1 medium pear
12 walnut halves OR 6 walnuts in shell

m e n u # 7
1 hot cross bun, split and toasted
2 tbsp (25 mL) fruit-flavoured light cream cheese
1/2 cup (125 mL) low-fat milk

m e n u # 8
1 weiner and roll
ketchup, relish and mustard
1/2 cup (125 mL) low-fat milk

m e n u #9	1 can (284 mL) ready-to-serve split pea soup 6 soda crackers
m e n u #10	1 **Raisin Bran Buttermilk Muffin** (page 49) 1 tsp (5 mL) soft margarine OR butter 1 cup (250 mL) low-fat milk
m e n u #11	3 tbsp (45 mL) **Curried Cheddar Spread** (page 182) 5 whole wheat soda crackers 1 medium apple
m e n u #12	2 cups (500 mL) **Popcorn Munch** (page 180) **Frosty Mocha Shake** *In blender container, combine 1/2 cup (125 mL) low-fat milk, 2 ice cubes, 1 tsp (5 mL) each: unsweetened cocoa powder and instant coffee granules, dash vanilla extract, sweetener to taste. Blend until smooth.*
m e n u #13	1 serving (1/12) warm **Homestyle Gingerbread** (page 121) 1/2 cup (125 mL) warm unsweetened applesauce 1 cup (250 mL) low-fat milk
m e n u #14	1 **Carrot Snacking Cake** (page 193) 1 cup (250 mL) low-fat milk
m e n u #15	1 serving (1/4) **Pineapple Upside-Down Cake** (page 194) 1/4 cup (50 mL) light vanilla ice cream

snack recipes index

PREPARATION TIME:
15 minutes

Each serving:
1/4 cup (50 mL)

1 PROTEIN CHOICE
1 EXTRA

3 g carbohydrate (0 g fibre)
6 g protein
3 g total fat (1 g saturated fat)
218 mg sodium
57 calories

75-calorie snack menu #10
150-calorie snack menu #20

Salsa Cheese Spread

A commercial salsa adds zesty flavour and moisture to this high-protein cheese spread. Adding carrot makes it an excellent source of vitamin A. Served with raw veggies or crackers, it becomes a great party appetizer.

1 cup	light (1%) cottage cheese	250 mL
1/2 cup	shredded light Cheddar cheese	125 mL
1/4 cup	mild OR medium salsa	50 mL
1 tbsp	light mayonnaise	15 mL
2 tsp	Dijon-style mustard	10 mL
1	medium carrot, grated (1/2 cup/125 mL)	1
1	green onion, chopped	1
1 tbsp	chopped fresh chives OR parsley	15 mL

1 Combine cottage cheese, Cheddar cheese, salsa, mayonnaise and mustard in food processor or blender. Process until smooth. Remove to bowl, stir in carrot, onion and chives.

2 Cover and refrigerate for at least 1 hour to allow flavours to develop. Keep for up to one week in the refrigerator or freeze for longer storage.

Makes about 2 cups (500 mL).

75-calorie snack menu #11

150-calorie snack menu #19

Frozen Melon Smoothie

Enjoy the sweet fruity flavour of cantaloupe in this elegant and healthy fruit drink. Of all the melons, cantaloupe is the highest in beta-carotene, potassium and vitamin C (see Tip). Garnish each serving with a lime slice or fresh mint sprig.

1/4 cup	low-fat (2%) evaporated milk	50 mL
1 1/2 cups	cubed ripe cantaloupe (see Tip)	375 mL
2 tsp	low-calorie sweetener	10 mL
1/2 cup	light vanilla ice cream	125 mL
4	ice cubes	4
	Lime slice OR fresh mint sprig	

1 Freeze milk in shallow metal bowl. Remove from freezer and transfer to blender container or food processor.

2 Add melon, sweetener, ice cream and ice cubes. Blend on high speed until slushy. Pour into 2 glasses and serve with lime or mint.

Makes 2 servings, about 2 cups (500 mL).

PREPARATION TIME:
20 minutes

Each serving:
1 cup (250 mL)

1 FRUITS & VEGETABLES CHOICE
1/2 SUGARS CHOICE
1 MILK 2% CHOICE

23 g carbohydrate (1 g fibre)
5 g protein
3 g total fat (2 g saturated fat)
75 mg sodium
138 calories

KITCHEN TIPS

Any of the bright orange and red fruits and vegetables, such as cantaloupe, mangoes, oranges, carrots, red pepper and squash are bursting with the antioxidants vitamin C and beta-carotene, which the body converts to vitamin A.

Since melons will not ripen further once they have been picked, be sure to choose a ripe one. A fruity fragrance, as well as a slight indentation in the stem end, may be a clue to maturity.

PREPARATION TIME:
10 minutes

COOKING TIME:
about 35 minutes

Each serving:
1 cup (250 mL)

1 STARCH CHOICE
1 FATS & OILS CHOICE

19 g carbohydrate (2 g fibre)
3 g protein
4 g total fat (1 g saturated fat)
307 mg sodium
120 calories

KITCHEN TIP

To air-pop, use an automatic corn popper or heat a large nonstick saucepan or electric skillet on medium-high heat for several minutes. Add about 1/2 cup (125 mL) unpopped kernels; shake pan until all kernels are popped. Cool, then measure the required 8 cups (2 L).

Variations

Try these interesting flavour variations:

• **Italian flavours**—dried oregano, basil and garlic powder

• **sweet seasonings**—ground cinnamon, nutmeg and cloves

• **hot 'n spicy**—dry mustard, hot sauce and paprika

75-calorie snack menu #12

150-calorie snack menu #28
300-calorie snack menu #13

Popcorn Munch

This snack is much more interesting than potato or tortilla chips and much lower in fat.

8 cups	air-popped corn (1/2 cup/125 mL kernels) (see Tip)	2 L
2 cups	small shredded wheat cereal squares	500 mL
1 1/4 cups	broken slim pretzels	300 mL
3 tbsp	melted soft margarine OR butter	45 mL
2 tbsp	freshly grated Parmesan cheese	25 mL
1 tsp	chili powder	5 mL
1/2 tsp	each: garlic powder and celery salt	2 mL

1 In plastic bag, combine cool air-popped corn, cereal and pretzels.

2 In small bowl, stir together margarine, cheese, chili powder, garlic powder and celery salt; pour over popped corn mixture in bag; shake well to distribute.

3 Spread on large baking pan. Bake in 275°F (140°C) oven for about 35 minutes or until golden brown and crispy. Cool before storing in airtight container or small sandwich bags.

Makes 11 cups (2.75 mL).

75-calorie snack menu #13
150-calorie snack menu #33
lunch menu #16

Pita Cheese Crisps

Kids and adults love these crispy low-fat snackers. Enjoy them as dippers for a snack or with soup. Change seasonings to suit your individual taste.

5	whole wheat pita breads (310 g total)	5
1/2 cup	freshly grated Parmesan cheese	125 mL
1 tsp	each: paprika, dried oregano and basil	5 mL
1/4 tsp	garlic powder	1 mL

1 With kitchen scissors, cut pita rounds in half and then separate. Lightly spray inside surface of each piece with nonstick vegetable spray.

2 In small bowl, combine cheese, paprika, oregano, basil and garlic powder. Distribute about 2 tsp (10 mL) over each pita half. With scissors, cut each half into 4 triangles. Arrange in single layer on large baking pan.

3 Bake in 300°F (160°C) oven for 15 minutes or until crisp and golden. Cool completely and store in tightly sealed container.

Makes 40 pieces.

PREPARATION TIME:
15 minutes

COOKING TIME:
15 to 18 minutes

Each serving:
4 pieces

1 STARCH CHOICE
1/2 PROTEIN CHOICE

17 g carbohydrate (0 g fibre)
5 g protein
2 g total fat (1 g saturated fat)
186 mg sodium
108 calories

PREPARATION TIME:
15 minutes

CHILL:
1 hour or longer

Each serving:
3 tbsp (45 mL)

1 PROTEIN CHOICE
1 FATS & OILS CHOICE
1 EXTRA

3 g carbohydrate (0 g fibre)
6 g protein
10 g total fat (4 g saturated fat)
269 mg sodium
117 calories

KITCHEN TIP

Line a bowl or mold with plastic wrap; pack the spread in the lined bowl, cover and refrigerate until firm. Cut into smaller pieces and freeze for longer storage.

75-calorie snack menu #16
150-calorie snack menu #24
300-calorie snack menu #12

Curried Cheddar Spread

This "nippy" spread served with crackers makes a delicious snack when a meal is delayed.

1 1/2 cups	shredded low-fat Cheddar cheese	375 mL
1/2 cup	light cream cheese (one-half 250 g pkg)	125 mL
1/2 cup	light mayonnaise	125 mL
2 tbsp	fruit chutney	25 mL
2 tsp	horseradish	10 mL
1 tsp	curry powder	5 mL
1/2 tsp	Worcestershire sauce	2 mL
Pinch	cayenne pepper	Pinch
1/4 cup	chopped parsley	50 mL
2 tbsp	finely chopped onion	25 mL

1 In food processor or blender, combine Cheddar cheese, cream cheese, mayonnaise, chutney, horseradish, curry powder, Worcestershire sauce and cayenne; process until smooth. Remove to bowl; stir in parsley and onion.

2 Refrigerate in tightly sealed container for up to one week or freeze for longer storage (see Tip).

Makes about 10 servings OR 2 cups (500 mL).

150-calorie snack menu #14

Buttermilk Scones

This hearty Scottish snack is cut into traditional wedge shapes. **Multimix** makes preparation quick and easy.

2 cups	**Multimix** (page 36)	500 mL
2 tbsp	dried currants OR raisins	25 mL
1 tbsp	granulated sugar	15 mL
1/2 cup	buttermilk or sour milk	125 mL
1	egg, beaten OR 2 egg whites	1
1 tsp	grated orange rind (optional)	5 mL
2 tbsp	all purpose flour	25 mL

1 In medium bowl, combine **Multimix**, currants and sugar.

2 In second bowl, stir together buttermilk, egg and orange rind. Pour into dry mixture; stir with fork until dry ingredients are just moistened.

3 Turn dough out onto lightly floured surface; knead gently about 20 times. Divide in two. Pat each piece into 6-inch (15 cm) round, about 1/2-inch (1 cm) thick. Transfer to ungreased baking sheet; cut each round with a knife into 6 triangles.

4 Bake in 375°F (190°C) oven for about 20 minutes or until lightly browned.

Makes 12 scones.

PREPARATION TIME:
15 minutes

COOKING TIME:
about 20 minutes

Each serving:
1 scone

1 STARCH CHOICE
1 FATS & OILS CHOICE

15 g carbohydrate (1 g fibre)
3 g protein
6 g fat (1 g saturated fat)
68 mg sodium
118 calories

PREPARATION TIME:
10 minutes

CHILL:
1 hour

Each serving:
1/4 cup (50 mL)

1 PROTEIN CHOICE

2 g carbohydrate (0 g fibre)
6 g protein
2 g total fat (1 g saturated fat)
323 mg sodium
52 calories

KITCHEN TIP

Great as a topping for baked potato.

150-calorie snack menu #15
Light Herb Cheese Spread

Cottage cheese with a difference! Keep this handy snacking spread in the refrigerator for up to one week.

1 cup	low-fat (1%) cottage cheese	250 mL
1 tbsp	light mayonnaise	15 mL
1 tbsp	cider vinegar	15 mL
2 tbsp	finely chopped parsley OR cilantro	25 mL
1	green onion, finely chopped	1
1/2 tsp	dried dill weed	2 mL
1/2 tsp	Dijon mustard	2 mL
1/4 tsp	salt	1 mL
Dash	hot pepper sauce	Dash

1 In blender or food processor, combine cottage cheese, mayonnaise and vinegar; process until smooth. Remove to bowl and stir in parsley, onion, dill weed, mustard, salt and hot pepper sauce.

2 Cover and refrigerate for at least 1 hour to allow flavours to develop. Keep for up to one week in the refrigerator or freeze for longer storage. (See Tip.)

Makes 1 1/2 cups (375 mL).

150-calorie snack menu #16
special occasions menu # 4

Multimix Tea Biscuits

Fast and easy to make with **Multimix** (page 36), these biscuits may be used for fruit shortcake or as a snack with a cup of tea.

2/3 cup	skim milk	150 mL
2 cups	**Multimix** (page 36)	500 mL
1 tbsp	all purpose flour	15 mL

1 In bowl, stir milk into **Multimix** with a fork just until dry ingredients are combined.

2 Turn out onto board lightly dusted with 1 tbsp (15 mL) flour; knead dough 20 times or until smooth. Roll dough to 1/2-inch (1 cm) thick. Cut 12 rounds with floured 2-inch (5 cm) biscuit cutter. Transfer to ungreased baking sheet.

3 Bake in 425°F (220°C) oven for about 12 minutes or until lightly browned.

Makes 12 biscuits.

PREPARATION TIME:
10 minutes

COOKING TIME:
about 12 minutes

Each serving:
1 biscuit

1 STARCH CHOICE
1 FATS & OILS CHOICE

12 g carbohydrate (1 g fibre)
2 g protein
5 g total fat (1 g saturated fat)
59 mg sodium
101 calories

PREPARATION TIME:
15 minutes

COOKING TIME:
10 minutes

Each serving:
2 cookies

1/2 STARCH CHOICE
1 FRUITS & VEGETABLES CHOICE
1/2 FATS & OILS CHOICE

17 g carbohydrate (1 g fibre)
3 g protein
3 g total fat (1 g saturated fat)
108 mg sodium
100 calories

KITCHEN TIP

To ensure that cookies are similar in size, use 2 teaspoons, one to scoop, the other to remove from spoon to baking pan.

150-calorie snack menu #21
Date 'n Raisin Soft Cookies

The joy of cookies! Peanut butter, rich in monounsaturated fat, replaces more saturated shortening or butter in this recipe. It also adds body, taste and texture. And rolled oats, our favourite grain, add fibre as well as a pleasant nutty flavour.

1/3 cup	chopped, packed raisins	75 mL
1/3 cup	chopped, packed dates	75 mL
1/2 cup	mashed banana (1 small)	125 mL
1/4 cup	creamy light peanut butter	50 mL
1/4 cup	water	50 mL
1	egg, beaten OR 2 egg whites	1
1 tsp	vanilla extract	5 mL
1 cup	quick-cooking rolled oats	250 mL
1/2 cup	all purpose flour	125 mL
1 tsp	baking soda	5 mL

1 In medium bowl, combine raisins, dates, banana, peanut butter, water, egg and vanilla. Stir in oats, flour and baking soda; blend well.

2 Drop by spoonfuls (see Tip) onto lightly greased or nonstick baking sheets; flatten with fork.

3 Bake in 350°F (180°C) oven for 10 minutes or until lightly browned. Cool completely on wire rack. Store in closed container.

Makes 30 cookies.

150-calorie snack menu #22

Hummus Dip with Tortilla Snackers

This high-fibre vegetarian dip is of Middle Eastern origin. It's East-West fusion when served with tortillas, the bread of Mexico.

Hummus

1	can (19 oz/540 mL) chick peas, drained	1
1 to 2	cloves garlic, minced	1 to 2
1/2 cup	low-fat (1%) plain yogurt	125 mL
3 tbsp	lemon juice	45 mL
1/2 tsp	salt	2 mL
1/2 tsp	ground cumin	2 mL
Dash	hot pepper sauce	Dash
	Freshly ground pepper	

Tortilla Snackers

4	8-inch (20 cm) flour tortillas (see Tip)	4

1 **Hummus:** In food processor or blender, purée chick peas with garlic until coarsely chopped. Add yogurt, lemon juice and seasonings; blend to a smooth paste.

2 Remove and refrigerate, covered, for at least 2 hours so flavours develop.

PREPARATION TIME:
10 minutes

CHILL:
2 hours or longer

Each serving:
1/3 cup (75 mL) Hummus with 6 Tortilla Snackers

1 1/2 STARCH CHOICES
1 PROTEIN CHOICE

28 g carbohydrate (4 g fibre)
7 g protein
3 g total fat (0 g saturated fat)
308 mg sodium
162 calories

KITCHEN TIPS

Freeze **Hummus Dip** in small amounts for later use, for dipping or as a sandwich spread.

Since flour tortillas come in packages of 10 or 12, bake extra snackers and keep in tightly closed container.

3 **Tortilla Snackers:** Cut each tortilla with scissors into 12 triangles. Place in single layer on baking pan. Bake in 300°F (150°C) oven for 15 to 20 minutes or until crisp and golden. Allow snackers to cool; store in tightly closed container (see Tip).

Makes 2 1/3 cups (575 mL) hummus and 48 tortilla snackers.

PREPARATION TIME:
10 minutes

COOKING TIME:
45 minutes

Each serving:
1/2 cup (125 mL)

1 STARCH CHOICE
1 FATS & OILS CHOICE

16 g carbohydrate (2 g fibre)
3 g protein
6 g total fat (1 g saturated fat)
307 mg sodium
123 calories

Snack Scramble

A tasty nibble to enjoy in the evening with cards or the news or to share with friends.

3 cups	small shredded wheat squares	750 mL
3 cups	O-shaped toasted oat cereal	750 mL
2 cups	slim pretzels	500 mL
1 cup	unsalted peanuts	250 mL
1/4 cup	melted soft margarine OR butter	50 mL
1 tbsp	Worcestershire sauce	15 mL
1 tsp	seasoned salt	5 mL
1/2 tsp	garlic powder	2 mL
Dash	hot pepper sauce	Dash

1 In large bowl, combine cereals, pretzels and peanuts. Stir together melted margarine, Worcestershire sauce, seasoned salt, garlic powder and hot pepper sauce. Pour over cereal mixture and toss to coat well.

2 Place mixture on large baking pan or roaster and bake in 250°F (125°C) oven for 45 minutes; stir every 15 minutes. Cool before storing in a tightly covered container.

Makes 18 servings, 9 cups (2.25 L).

150-calorie snack menu #29
Bagel Thins

It's great that bagels are low in fat because they taste so good. This recipe gives us thin slices pepped up with interesting seasonings. It's also a way to revamp stale bagels.

3	bagels (90 g each)	3
2 tbsp	olive oil	25 mL
	Garlic powder, seasoned salt, Italian herbs, sesame OR poppy seeds	

1 Slice each bagel in half to form semicircle. With very sharp bread knife, slice each semicircle horizontally into 6 thin slices, about 1/8-inch (5 mm). Arrange on baking pan; brush each bagel lightly with oil. Sprinkle with choice of seasonings.

2 Bake in 400°F (200°C) oven for 8 minutes or until golden brown and crisp. Cool and store in a tightly closed container for several weeks.

Makes 36 bagel thins.

PREPARATION TIME:
15 minutes

COOKING TIME:
8 to 10 minutes

Each serving:
4 slices

1 STARCH CHOICE
1/2 FATS & OILS CHOICE

17 g carbohydrate (0 g fibre)
3 g protein
3 g total fat (0 g saturated fat)
275 mg sodium
108 calories

PREPARATION TIME:
15 minutes

COOKING TIME:
9 minutes

Each serving:
2 cookies

1/2 STARCH CHOICE
1/2 FRUITS & VEGETABLES
CHOICE
1/2 SUGARS CHOICE
1 FATS & OILS CHOICE

18 g carbohydrate (1 g fibre)
2 g protein
4 g total fat (1 g saturated fat)
107 mg sodium
114 calories

150-calorie snack menu #30
Carrot Raisin Oat Cookies

Great at munch-time with a cup of light hot chocolate or a glass of milk, these cookies are full of the good nutrition of carrots and oats.

1/2 cup	firmly packed brown sugar	125 mL
1/3 cup	soft margarine OR butter	75 mL
1	egg OR 2 egg whites	1
1 tsp	vanilla extract	5 mL
1 cup	finely shredded carrots (2 medium)	250 mL
1/4 cup	raisins, chopped	50 mL
1 cup	large flake rolled oats	250 mL
1 cup	all purpose flour	250 mL
1/2 cup	granular low-calorie sweetener with sucralose	125 mL
2 1/2 tsp	baking powder	12 mL
1/2 tsp	ground cinnamon	2 mL
1/4 tsp	each: ground nutmeg and salt	1 mL

1 In large bowl, combine sugar, margarine, egg and vanilla; beat well. Stir in carrots and raisins. Add oats, flour, sweetener, baking powder, cinnamon, nutmeg and salt; stir to blend well.

2 Lightly spray large baking sheets with nonstick vegetable coating. Drop batter by spoonfuls onto pans; flatten with fork.

3 Bake in 375°F (190°C) oven for 9 minutes or until lightly browned. Cool completely on wire rack. Store in tightly closed container.

Makes 36 cookies.

150-calorie snack menu #31

Cranberry Scones

The refreshing cranberry-orange flavour of these **Multimix**-based scones is superb with a cup of tea.

1 tsp	granulated sugar	5 mL
1/4 tsp	each: ground ginger and nutmeg	1 mL
2 cups	**Multimix** (page 36)	500 mL
1/2 cup	chopped fresh or frozen cranberries	125 mL
1 tbsp	granulated sugar	15 mL
1 tbsp	grated orange zest	15 mL
1/2 cup	buttermilk or sour milk	125 mL
1	egg, beaten OR 2 egg whites	1
2 tbsp	all purpose flour	25 mL

1 Combine sugar, ginger and nutmeg; set aside.

2 In medium bowl, combine **Multimix**, cranberries, sugar and orange zest.

3 Stir together buttermilk and egg. Add to dry ingredients, stirring with fork just until moistened.

4 Lightly dust board with 2 tbsp (25 mL) flour; knead dough gently on board about 20 times or until smooth. Roll dough about 1/2-inch (1 cm) thick; cut with 3-inch (7.5 cm) cutter. Place on ungreased baking sheet.

5 Bake in 375°F (190°C) oven for 20 minutes or until lightly browned.

Makes 10 scones.

PREPARATION TIME:
15 minutes

COOKING TIME:
about 20 minutes

Each serving:
1 scone

**1 STARCH CHOICE
1 1/2 FATS & OILS CHOICES**

16 g carbohydrate (1 g fibre)
3 g protein
7 g total fat (2 g saturated fat)
75 mg sodium
134 calories

KITCHEN TIP

Increased availability of dried cranberries, cherries and, yes, even blueberries, allows us to make these scones year-round. Replace 1/2 cup (125 mL) fresh cranberries with 2 tbsp (25 mL) of any of these dried fruits.

Garden Tomato Salsa

PREPARATION TIME:
10 minutes

CHILL:
at least 30 minutes

Each serving:
1/4 cup (50 mL)

1 EXTRA

3 g carbohydrate (1 g fibre)
0 g protein
0 g fat
95 mg sodium
11 calories

Variation: Salsa and Cheese Dip

Stir together 1/3 cup (75 mL) each:
light ricotta cheese and **Garden
Tomato Salsa**.

Makes 2 servings.

Salsa and Cheese Dip:
Each serving:
1/3 cup (75 mL)

**1 PROTEIN CHOICE
1 EXTRA**

4 g carbohydrate (1 g fibre)
5 g protein
3 g total fat (2 g saturated fat)
114 mg sodium
64 calories

This versatile condiment is much lower in sodium than commercial ones. Use it alone or with ricotta cheese (see below) to dip tortilla chips. Pep up baked beans, scrambled eggs and meats with its spicy tomato fresh flavours.

1 1/2 cups	chopped tomatoes (2 medium)	375 mL
1	jalapeño pepper, seeded and chopped (see Tip)	1
1/3 cup	diced sweet red pepper	75 mL
1/4 cup	chopped fresh cilantro (see Tip)	50 mL
2 tbsp	finely chopped onion	25 mL
2	cloves garlic, crushed	2
2 tbsp	balsamic vinegar	25 mL
1/4 tsp	each: salt and freshly ground pepper	1 mL

1 In bowl, combine tomatoes, jalapeño and red pepper, cilantro, onion and garlic; stir in vinegar, salt and pepper. Cover and refrigerate for at least 30 minutes.

Makes 2 cups (500 mL).

KITCHEN TIPS

Use either fresh or pickled jalapeños, whichever are available.

If fresh cilantro (sometimes called coriander or Chinese parsley) is not available, replace with 1/4 cup (50 mL) chopped fresh parsley and 1 tsp (5 mL) dried coriander.

Keeps well in the refrigerator for up to one week.

300-calorie snack menu #15

Carrot Snacking Cake

When **Make-Ahead Double Bran Muffin Batter** (page 45) is sitting in your refrigerator, turn part of it into carrot cake. Only 1/6 of the batter makes 3 servings, leaving enough for muffins! Carrots add texture and moisture to this traditional cake.

1 cup	**Make-Ahead Double Bran Muffin Batter**	250 mL
1/4 cup	shredded carrots	50 mL
1/2 tsp	vanilla extract	2 mL

1 Spray three 3/4 cup (175 mL) custard cups with non-stick vegetable coating.

2 In medium bowl, gently stir together batter, carrots and vanilla extract. Divide batter evenly between cups.

3 Bake in 350°F (180°C) oven for 20 minutes or until top springs back when lightly touched. Cool for 5 minutes. Remove from cups to wire rack to cool.

Makes 3 cakes.

PREPARATION TIME:
5 minutes (with prepared batter)

COOKING TIME:
20 minutes

Each serving:
1 cake

1 STARCH CHOICE
1 SUGARS CHOICE
1/2 PROTEIN CHOICE
1 FATS & OILS CHOICE

28 g carbohydrate (4 g fibre)
5 g protein
8 g total fat (1 g saturated fat)
273 mg sodium
192 calories

PREPARATION TIME:
5 minutes with prepared batter

COOKING TIME:
25 minutes

Each serving:
1 slice

1/2 STARCH CHOICE
1 FRUITS & VEGETABLES CHOICE
1 SUGARS CHOICE
1/2 PROTEIN CHOICE
1 1/2 FATS & OILS CHOICES

33 g carbohydrate (3 g fibre)
4 g protein
9 g total fat (1 g saturated fat)
242 mg sodium
215 calories

300-calorie snack menu #16
Pineapple Upside Down Cake

Served right side up or upside down, warm or cold, the fresh tropical flavour of pineapple makes this snack special. It's easy and quickly made using our **Make-Ahead Double Bran Muffin Batter** (page 45) One slice is a high source of fibre.

1 tbsp	soft margarine OR butter	15 mL
1 tbsp	brown sugar	15 mL
1 tbsp	granulated brown low-calorie sweetener	15 mL
4	pineapple slices	4
4	dried sweetened cranberries	4
1 cup	**Make-Ahead Double Bran Muffin Batter**	250 mL

1 Spray 8-inch (20 cm) round cake pan with non-stick vegetable coating.

2 Melt margarine in pan. Stir in brown sugar and sweetener. Place pineapple rings over mixture; place 1 dried cranberry in each hole. Spoon muffin batter over pineapple. Bake in 350°F (180°C) oven for 25 minutes or until top springs back when lightly touched. Serve warm or cold.

Makes 4 servings.

special occasions

Anniversaries, birthdays, retirements, reunions! Commemorate these special occasions with an at-home gathering. The six menus in this section are for entertaining in your home, perhaps with your family, maybe with good friends. Special occasions most often involve guests, so we have designed this chapter's recipes and menus for four to six people. Some menus are for specific occasions—a brunch, a summer picnic or a holiday get-together. Other menus include a **Greek Taverna Dinner** (page 197) and **Puttin' on the Ritz** (page 197).

Naturally these meals require a bit more preparation time than our regular day-to-day menus, but they are, after all, for special occasions. Several are higher in fat and sodium than our usual menus, but the carbohydrate content remains the same. Brunch is based on the Lunch meal plan, the others the Dinner plan (see page 15). After all, it's what you eat 80% of the time, not what you eat occasionally, that matters. All menus remain true to healthy eating goals and give suggested serving sizes for those watching their portions.

Eating Out

On other occasions you may be invited to someone's home. Not being in control of the menu doesn't have to be a problem for the person with diabetes. Just try to stay with your usual portions. Eat sparingly or leave items that don't fit your meal plan. A thoughtful host or hostess will inquire about your diet needs beforehand. Dining out at a restaurant—not a problem. At least you can make choices from the menu.

Non-Alcoholic Beverages for Special Occasions

Looking for an EXTRA low- or no-calorie thirst quencher? Try one of these:

- mineral water or soda water with lime
- water, clear tea, black coffee
- diet soft drinks
- iced tea with sweetener
- homemade lemonade with sweetener
- low-calorie drink mixes, alone or mixed with diet gingerale or diet 7Up™

Alcohol and Special Occasions

Special occasions often include an alcoholic drink before or with a meal. Current CDA guidelines consider one or two drinks per day acceptable as long as there are no other problems such as elevated cholesterol or triglyceride levels or hypertension. If you are taking insulin or diabetes pills or other medications, discuss the use of alcohol with your diabetes health care team first.

Tips to Remember

- Always eat food when drinking alcohol. Never drink on an empty stomach.

- Alcohol can cause hypoglycemia or low blood sugar (see page 224) if you are on insulin or certain diabetes medications. Learn how to recognize symptoms (cold, sweating, shaking, very hungry), how to treat it (glucose candies or juice) and, better still, how to prevent it.

- Alcohol has extra calories. If you are watching your weight, remember that one average drink can add 100 to 150 extra calories to your meal.

- Here is a comparison of some drinks, their food choice values and their calorie content.

Type of Drink	Amount	Food Choice Value	Energy Value in Calories
dry red or white wine	3.5 oz (100 mL)	1 1/2 FATS & OILS	63
whiskey, rye, gin, Scotch, vodka, rum, brandy, cognac	1.5 oz (45 mL)	2 FATS & OILS	105
dry sherry	2 oz (60 mL)	1 1/2 FATS & OILS	63
regular beer	12 oz (340 mL)	1 STARCH + 2 FATS & OILS	150
light beer	12 oz (340 mL)	1/2 STARCH + 1 1/2 FATS & OILS	112

Source: Good Health Eating Guide Resource (1999), Canadian Diabetes Association, with permission.

menus for special occasions

special occasion menu #1

Puttin' on the Ritz, serves 8
(with amounts for one serving)

1 cup (250 mL) **Spicy Tomato Wine Bouillon** (page 201)

1 chop from **Crown Roast of Pork** with
1/2 cup (125 mL) **Wild Rice Almond Dressing** (page 202)

1/8 **Balsamic Baked Mushrooms** (page 204)

1 cup (250 mL) green beans
1 tbsp (15 mL) chopped sweet red pepper

1/8 **Fruits aux Chocolat** (page 206)

tea or coffee

special occasion menu #2

Greek Taverna Dinner, serves 6
(with amounts for one serving)

1/4 cup (50 mL) **Tzatsiki Appetizer** (page 208)
with 1/2 pita bread (30 g)

1/6 **Moussaka** (page 209)

1/6 **Marouli Salata** (page 210)

1 small orange, sliced; sprinkled with ground cinnamon

tea or coffee

special occasion menu #3

Brunch Time, serves 6 or 12
(with amounts for one serving)

1/6 **Peaches 'n Blueberries French Toast** (page 211)

1/4 cup (50 mL) **Peach-Blueberry Fruit Sauce** (page 212)

1 slice (25 g) Canadian back bacon

1 **Ginger Bran Muffin** (page 50)

2/3 cup (150 mL) **Sunrise Mimosa** (page 212)

tea or coffee

special occasion menu #4

Gourmet Dinner, serves 4 to 6
(with amounts for one serving)

1 cup (250 mL) **Rhubarb Punch** (page 213)
1/3 cup (75 mL) concentrate with soda water and ice

1 **Poached Chicken Breast** (page 214) with
3 tbsp (45 mL) **Cranberry Coulis** (page 215)

1/2 cup (125 mL) **Barley Pilaf** (page 216)

1/2 cup (125 mL) steamed green beans
with 1 tsp (5 mL) toasted slivered almonds

1/6 **Favourite Caesar Salad** (page 133)

1/6 **Strawberry Shortcake** (page 217)

tea or coffee

special occasion menu #5

A Summer Picnic, serves 6
(with amounts for one serving)

2 pieces **Crispy Baked Chicken** (page 218)

1/2 cup (125 mL) **Summertime Potato Salad** (page 124)

1/2 cup (125 mL) coleslaw with oil and vinegar

assorted raw vegetables: *celery sticks, zucchini sticks, cucumber slices, green onions, radishes, cherry tomatoes* with 1/3 cup (75 mL) **Creamy Herb Dip** (page 219)

1 large peach

fruit-flavored sugar-free mineral water

special occasion menu #6

Holiday Dinner, serves 6
(with amounts for one serving)

1 cup (250 mL) consommé with chopped parsley

3 slices (90 g) chicken OR roast turkey

2/3 cup (150 mL) **Poultry Dressing** (page 220)
1/4 cup (50 mL) **Light Gravy** (page 119)

1/2 cup (125 mL) mashed potatoes

1 cup (250 mL) French-style green beans

1/2 cup (125 mL) **Braised Red Cabbage with Cranberries** (page 221)

Raspberry Parfait
*3 tbsp (45 mL) **Raspberry Sauce** (page 222)
over 1/3 cup (75 mL) light vanilla ice cream*

tea or coffee

special occasions recipes index

special occasions recipes

Spicy Tomato Wine Bouillon

This light soup excites the taste buds in anticipation of the elegant meal to follow, yet adds few calories.

4 cups	tomato juice	1 L
3 cups	beef broth	750 mL
1/2 cup	chopped onion	125 mL
3	sprigs fresh parsley	3
1 tbsp	granular low-calorie sweetener with sucralose	15 mL
1/4 tsp	freshly ground pepper	1 mL
2	whole cloves	2
1 cup	dry white OR red wine (see Tip)	250 mL
1/4 cup	dry sherry	50 mL
1	lemon, thinly sliced	1
	Paprika	

1 In large saucepan, combine tomato juice, broth, onion, parsley, sweetener, pepper and cloves; bring to boil. Reduce heat, cover and simmer for 30 minutes. Strain and return to saucepan. Add wine and sherry and heat to serving temperature. Serve with lemon slices sprinkled with paprika.

Makes 8 servings, 8 cups (2 L).

PREPARATION TIME:
10 minutes

COOKING TIME:
about 30 minutes

Each serving:
1 cup (250 mL)

1/2 FRUITS & VEGETABLES CHOICE
1/2 FATS & OILS CHOICE
1 EXTRA

8 g carbohydrate (1 g fibre)
2 g protein
0 g total fat
426 mg sodium
61 calories

KITCHEN TIP

When cooking with wine, always add it half way through the cooking time so the flavours are not boiled away. Alcohol evaporates when wine is simmered. All you are left with is the superb taste. If you wish to omit the wine and sherry, replace with extra broth.

PREPARATION TIME:
15 minutes

COOKING TIME:
about 3 1/2 hours

Each serving:
1 chop and 1/2 cup (125 mL) dressing

1/2 STARCH CHOICE
3 1/2 PROTEIN CHOICES
1 EXTRA

13 g carbohydrate (2 g fibre)
26 g protein
10 g total fat (3 g saturated fat)
152 mg sodium
243 calories

special occasions menu #1

Crown Roast of Pork with Wild Rice Almond Dressing

For that ritzy occasion, what is more spectacular than a lean, gourmet crown roast of pork with a wild rice dressing? Have your butcher partially cut the rib bones to make carving easier. Leftovers will be superb.

7 lb	lean crown roast of pork (14 to 16 chops)	3 kg

Dressing

1 cup	wild rice	250 mL
2	bay leaves	2
2 tsp	soft margarine OR butter	10 mL
2 cups	sliced mushrooms (about 12 small)	500 mL
1 cup	chopped onion (about 1 large)	250 mL
1 cup	thinly sliced celery	250 mL
6	slices whole wheat bread	6
1/3 cup	slivered almonds, toasted	75 mL
1/4 cup	chopped fresh parsley	50 mL
1 tsp	dried thyme OR 1 tbsp (15 mL) fresh	5 mL
1/2 tsp	each: salt, freshly ground black pepper and dried summer savory	2 mL

1 Place meat on rack in a shallow pan. Wrap rib bones with foil. Stuff ball of foil in middle to keep cavity open. Roast, uncovered, in 325°F (160°C) oven for 2 hours.

special occasions menu #1

2 Meanwhile, wash wild rice thoroughly under cold running water. In medium saucepan, bring 3 cups (750 mL) water to boil. Add rice and bay leaves, reduce heat, cover and simmer for 45 minutes or until rice is tender; drain and discard bay leaves.

3 In large nonstick skillet, melt margarine over medium-high heat; cook mushrooms, onion and celery for 6 minutes or until tender. Stir into rice. Crumble bread crumbs. Stir crumbs, almonds, parsley, thyme, salt, pepper and savory into onion mixture.

4 Remove roast from oven, remove foil; fill centre with some dressing. Cover dressing with small piece of foil. Place remaining dressing in casserole (see Kitchen Tip for cooking directions).

5 Place meat thermometer in thickest part of meat, not touching bone. Roast an additional 3/4 to 1 1/2 hours or until thermometer registers 160°F (70°C). Place meat on carving platter. Allow to rest for 10 minutes before carving. Remove foil from dressing. Slice between ribs to serve.

Makes 14 to 16 chops and about 9 cups (2.25 L) dressing.

KITCHEN TIP

There will not be enough room for all the dressing in the centre of the roast. Place the extra in a casserole lightly sprayed with nonstick vegetable coating. Cook alongside roast for about 1 hour or until heated and golden.

PREPARATION TIME:
10 minutes

COOKING TIME:
15 minutes

Each serving:
1/8 of recipe

1/2 FRUITS & VEGETABLES CHOICE
1 FATS & OILS

7 g carbohydrate (2 g fibre)
3 g protein
4 g total fat (1 g saturated fat)
37 mg sodium
65 calories

Balsamic Baked Mushrooms

This wonderful, unique low-fat vegetable recipe is an excellent accompaniment to roast pork, chicken or turkey. The mushrooms also barbecue well placed on the rack above grilling meats.

9 cups	thickly sliced mushrooms (2 lb/900 g)	2.25 L
3/4 cup	thinly sliced onions (2 small)	175 mL
1/2 cup	**Balsamic Vinaigrette Dressing** (page 205)	125 mL

1 Place mushrooms and onions in shallow baking pan. Drizzle with vinaigrette.

2 Bake, uncovered, in 375°F (190°C) oven for 20 minutes or until mushrooms are cooked.

Makes 8 servings.

special occasions menu #1
Balsamic Vinaigrette Dressing

Balsamic vinegar in a dressing imparts a wonderful flavour to tossed green salads, adding extra flavour to a vinaigrette. It is superb in the recipe for **Balsamic Baked Mushrooms** (page 204). Good balsamic vinegar is relatively costly, but the flavour delivery is well worth the price. A little goes a long way!

1/2 cup	balsamic vinegar	125 mL
1/3 cup	water	75 mL
2 tbsp	finely chopped red onion	25 mL
1 tsp	Dijon mustard	5 mL
1	clove garlic, finely minced	1
1 tsp	granular low-calorie sweetener with sucralose	5 mL
1/4 tsp	salt	1 mL
Pinch	freshly ground pepper	Pinch
1/4 cup	olive oil (see Tip)	50 mL

1 In small bowl, combine vinegar, water, onion, mustard, garlic, sweetener, salt and pepper. Whisk in oil until well blended. Pour into covered container and refrigerate until ready to use.

Makes about 1 cup (250 mL).

PREPARATION TIME:
5 minutes

CHILL:
until ready to use

Each serving:
1 tbsp (15 mL)

1/2 FATS & OILS CHOICE

1 g carbohydrate (0 g fibre)
0 g protein
3 g fat (0 g saturated fat)
34 mg sodium
32 calories

KITCHEN TIP

For a fat-free dressing, use chicken or beef stock to replace oil. Then 1 tbsp (15 mL) dressing may be considered an EXTRA.

PREPARATION TIME:
30 minutes

COOKING TIME:
about 5 minutes for the **Chocolate Fondue**

Each serving:
2 tbsp (25 mL) **Chocolate Fondue**, 1/3 cup (75 mL) cantaloupe cubes, 1/3 cup (75 mL) honeydew melon balls and 6 strawberries

2 FRUITS & VEGETABLES CHOICES
1/2 MILK 2% CHOICE
1/2 SUGARS CHOICE
1/2 FATS & OILS CHOICE

31 g carbohydrate (5 g fibre)
4 g protein
5 g total fat (2 g saturated fat)
109 mg sodium
168 calories

Fruits aux Chocolat

Dipping fruit into this wondrous chocolate sauce is a fine ending to a very special meal.

1 cup	**Chocolate Fondue** (page 207)	250 mL
2 2/3 cups	cantaloupe melon cubes	650 mL
2 2/3 cups	honeydew melon balls	650 mL
48	strawberries, halved	48

1 Warm chocolate sauce over hot but not boiling water. Remove to fondue pot to keep warm.

2 Meanwhile, prepare fruits. To serve, dip fruit pieces into warm sauce using wooden skewers.

Makes 8 servings.

special occasions menu #1

Chocolate Fondue

Many believe chocolate is the perfect finish for a meal. Satisfy this craving with chocolate sauce served over fresh fruit. We use cocoa instead of higher-fat chocolate.

1/4 cup	soft margarine OR butter	50 mL
1/2 cup	cocoa powder	125 mL
1/3 cup	corn syrup	75 mL
1 1/2 cups	low-fat evaporated milk	375 mL
4 tsp	cornstarch	20 mL
1/2 cup	granular low-calorie sweetener with sucralose	125 mL
2 tsp	vanilla OR rum extract	10 mL

1 In small saucepan, melt margarine over medium-low heat. Whisk in cocoa until smooth.

2 Combine corn syrup, milk and cornstarch. Gradually stir into cocoa mixture. Cook gently on low heat for 5 minutes or until bubbly and smooth; stir occasionally. Stir in sweetener and vanilla.

3 Cool before storing in covered container in refrigerator. Serve either cold or warm.

Makes 2 cups (500 mL).

PREPARATION TIME:
5 minutes

COOKING TIME:
about 10 minutes

Each serving:
2 tbsp (25 mL)

1/2 MILK 2% CHOICE
1/2 SUGARS CHOICE
1/2 FATS & OILS CHOICE

9 g carbohydrate (1 g fibre)
2 g protein
4 g total fat (3 g saturated fat)
54 mg sodium
75 calories

PREPARATION TIME:
10 minutes if yogurt is drained

CHILL:
up to 4 days

Each serving:
1/4 cup (50 mL)

1 MILK 2% CHOICE

6 g carbohydrate (0 g fibre)
4 g protein
1 g total fat (0 g saturated fat)
105 mg sodium
48 calories

KITCHEN TIPS

Check labels when choosing plain yogurt for yogurt cheese. Be sure to choose one without gelatin, starch or gums as they will not drain. Naturally, whole milk yogurts taste richest and are milder flavoured and smoother. Low- and non-fat yogurts are more tart with a tangy taste thus making a tangier yogurt cheese. Some people like to add the whey drained from yogurt to soups as it contains B vitamins and minerals.

To store yogurt cheese, cover and refrigerate for up to one week.

Yogurt cheese is also great for spreads, salad dressings, baked potatoes and can be a cream cheese replacement.

special occasions menu #2
Tzatziki Appetizer

This light and refreshing *mezé* (Greek for appetizer) is best made with drained yogurt, often referred to as yogurt cheese. You can adjust the garlic "hit" to suit your personal taste—more or less.

2 cups	low-fat (1%) plain yogurt (see Tip)	500 mL
1	small seedless cucumber, unpeeled, grated (about 2 cups/500 mL)	1
2	small cloves garlic, crushed	2
2 tsp	olive oil	10 mL
2 tsp	white vinegar	10 mL
1 tbsp	chopped fresh dill	15 mL
1/4 tsp	each: salt and pepper	1 mL

1 Line a sieve with cheesecloth or coffee filter paper; set over a medium bowl. Place yogurt in sieve. Cover and refrigerate for several hours or overnight. Gather edges of cheesecloth together and gently squeeze out any remaining whey liquid. Transfer yogurt cheese to a bowl.

2 Drain and squeeze liquid from cucumber. Stir cucumber, garlic, oil, vinegar, dill, salt and pepper into yogurt cheese. Cover and refrigerate until ready to serve. Stir just before serving.

Makes 8 servings, 2 cups (500 mL).

special occasions menu #2
Moussaka

There are as many versions of moussaka as there are Greek cooks. Traditional recipes sauté the eggplant in olive oil. Our way of baking the eggplant slices reduces fat, yet still retains the flavours of the traditional recipe.

2	large eggplants (1 lb/500 g each)	2
1 tsp	garlic powder	5 mL
1 lb	extra lean ground beef OR lamb	450 g
1/2 cup	chopped onion	125 mL
1	can (213 mL) tomato sauce	1
1/2 cup	dry red OR white wine OR chicken broth	125 mL
1/2 tsp	salt	2 mL
1/4 tsp	each: ground cloves, cinnamon, nutmeg and freshly ground pepper	1 mL

PREPARATION TIME:
30 minutes

COOKING TIME:
40 minutes

Each serving:
1/6 of recipe

1 1/2 FRUITS & VEGETABLES CHOICES
1 MILK 2% CHOICE
3 PROTEIN CHOICES

27 g carbohydrate (5 g fibre)
26 g protein
11 g total fat (2 g saturated fat)
513 mg sodium, 309 calories

White Sauce

1	can (385 mL) low-fat evaporated milk	1
1/2 cup	chicken broth	125 mL
1/4 cup	all purpose flour	50 mL
Pinch	white pepper	Pinch
1/4 cup	freshly grated Parmesan cheese	50 mL

1 Slice eggplant into 1/4-inch (6 mm) thick slices. Spray large baking sheets with nonstick coating. Place eggplant slices, not overlapping, on pan. Sprinkle with garlic powder. Bake in 425°F (220°C) oven for 15 minutes or until lightly browned. Set aside.

2 Meanwhile, in large nonstick skillet, cook beef over medium heat, stirring to break up, for 5 minutes or until all pink has disappeared; drain fat and discard. Return meat to skillet; add onion and cook for 5 minutes or until onions are tender. Add tomato sauce, wine, salt, cloves, cinnamon, nutmeg and pepper; simmer for 15 minutes, stirring occasionally.

3 **White Sauce:** In saucepan, whisk together milk, broth, flour and pepper. Cook over medium heat for 10 minutes or until smooth and thickened; stir frequently.

4 Lightly spray 11 × 7-inch (28 × 17 cm) baking pan with nonstick vegetable coating. Arrange 1/2 of eggplant in overlapping slices in bottom of pan. Top with 1/2 of sauce. Spread with 1/2 of meat mixture. Repeat layers; sprinkle with Parmesan cheese.

5 Cover and bake in 350°F (180°C) oven for 30 minutes; remove cover and cook for 10 minutes or until thoroughly heated.

Makes 6 servings.

PREPARATION TIME:
10 minutes

Each serving:
1/6 of recipe

1 FATS & OILS CHOICE
1 EXTRA

2 g carbohydrate (1 g fibre)
1 g protein
4 g total fat (1 g saturated fat)
44 mg sodium
45 calories

special occasions menu #2

Marouli Salata

Salata is the Greek word for salad and *marouli* means lettuce. Slicing the romaine lettuce as thinly as possible gives this very traditional salad its unique character.

1	medium head romaine lettuce, trimmed and washed	1
3	green onions, sliced	3
2 tbsp	chopped fresh dill	25 mL
2 tbsp	each: olive oil and lemon juice	25 mL
Pinch	each: salt and freshly ground black pepper	Pinch

1 Spin lettuce to dry. Roll 4 or 5 leaves tightly together; thinly slice with sharp knife. Repeat with remaining leaves until you have approximately 8 cups (2 L).

2 In a large salad bowl, combine lettuce, onions and dill. Just before serving, pour oil and lemon juice over and toss well. Sprinkle with salt and pepper.

Makes 6 servings.

special occasions menu #3

Peaches 'n Blueberries French Toast

This fruit version of the traditional strata is much lower in fat. It still provides the convenience of night-before preparation for weekend entertaining.

3/4 cup	light ricotta cheese	175 mL
4 tsp	granulated sugar	20 mL
4 tsp	granular low-calorie sweetener with sucralose	20 mL
2 tsp	grated orange rind	10 mL
1 tsp	vanilla extract	5 mL
3	eggs	3
1 1/4 cups	low-fat milk	300 mL
12	slices 1-inch (2.5 cm) thick French bread stick (180 g total)	12
2/3 cup	cubed fresh or frozen peaches	150 mL
1/2 cup	fresh or frozen blueberries	125 mL
	Ground nutmeg	

PREPARATION TIME:
15 minutes

COOKING TIME:
40 minutes

Each serving:
1/6 French Toast

1 STARCH CHOICE
1/2 SUGARS CHOICE
1 MILK 2% CHOICE
1 PROTEIN CHOICE
1/2 FATS & OILS CHOICE

28 g carbohydrate (1 g fibre)
11 g protein
7 g total fat (3 g saturated fat)
256 mg sodium
216 calories

1. In large bowl, blend ricotta cheese, sugar, sweetener, orange rind and vanilla until smooth. Add eggs and beat well. Stir in milk.

2. Lightly spray 11 × 7-inch (2 L) oblong baking pan with nonstick coating. Place bread slices upright in rows in pan. Pour egg mixture over bread, being careful to coat each slice. Top with peaches and blueberries; sprinkle with nutmeg. Cover and refrigerate for several hours or overnight.

3. Bake, uncovered, in 350°F (180°C) oven for 40 minutes or until golden brown and set in centre. Cut into 6 servings. Serve with **Peach-Blueberry Sauce** (page 212).

Makes 6 servings.

PREPARATION TIME:
10 minutes

COOKING TIME:
5 minutes

Each serving:
1/4 cup (50 mL)

1/2 FRUITS & VEGETABLES CHOICE

6 g carbohydrate (1 g fibre)
0 g protein
0 g total fat
2 mg sodium
25 calories

PREPARATION TIME:
5 minutes

CHILL:
1 to 2 hours

Each serving:
2/3 cup (150 mL)

1 FRUITS & VEGETABLES CHOICE

10 g carbohydrate (0 g fibre)
0 g protein
0 g total fat
18 mg sodium
36 calories

special occasions menu #3
Peach-Blueberry Fruit Sauce

Fresh and easily made, this fruit sauce complements **Peaches 'n Blueberries French Toast** (page 211). The sauce doubles the hit of these fresh fruits!

2/3 cup	water	150 mL
1/2 cup	cubed fresh or frozen peaches	125 mL
1/2 cup	fresh or frozen blueberries	125 mL
1 tbsp	each: granulated sugar and sweetener	15 mL
2 tsp	grated orange rind	10 mL
1 tsp	cornstarch	5 mL
Pinch	ground nutmeg	Pinch

1. In saucepan, combine water, peaches, blueberries, sugar, sweetener, orange rind, cornstarch and nutmeg. Cook on medium heat for 5 minutes or until slightly thickened and clear. Serve warm.

Makes 6 servings, 1 1/2 cups (375 mL) sauce.

Sunrise Mimosa

Equal parts orange juice and soda water (or champagne) served icy cold, but not over ice, makes this favourite brunch cocktail so good.

2 cups	orange juice, freshly squeezed	500 mL
2 cups	chilled soda water OR champagne	500 mL

1. Add orange juice to a large pitcher. Store in refrigerator. Just before serving, add soda water (or champagne). Serve at once.

Makes 6 servings, 4 cups (1 L).

special occasions menu #4
Rhubarb Punch

Tangy rhubarb makes this thirst-quenching beverage such a delight. Prepare concentrate in large amounts when spring rhubarb is available. Freeze in smaller amounts for use during the year.

4	oranges	4
2	lemons	2
8 cups	sliced fresh or frozen rhubarb	2 L
4 cups	water	1 L
1 cup	granular low-calorie sweetener with sucralose	250 mL

1 Remove rind from oranges and lemons. Squeeze juice and reserve.

2 In large saucepan, combine rhubarb, water, orange and lemon rind. Cover and cook over medium heat for 10 minutes or until rhubarb is tender.

3 Remove from heat; stir in lemon and orange juice. Cool. Press through a sieve to remove rhubarb pulp; discard pulp.

4 Add sweetener to strained juice. Pour into sterilized bottles and seal. Store in refrigerator or freeze for longer storage.

5 To serve: Combine 1/3 cup (75 mL) punch concentrate with 3/4 cup (175 mL) water, soda water or mineral water. Serve over ice cubes.

Makes 6 cups (1.5 L) punch concentrate.

PREPARATION TIME:
20 minutes

COOKING TIME:
about 10 minutes

Each serving:
1/3 cup (75 mL) concentrate

1/2 FRUITS & VEGETABLES CHOICE

6 g carbohydrate (1 g fibre)
1 g protein
0 g total fat
5 mg sodium
23 calories

PREPARATION TIME:
10 minutes

COOKING TIME:
15 minutes

Each serving:
1/2 chicken breast

3 PROTEIN CHOICES

0 g carbohydrate
27 g protein
3 g total fat (1 g saturated fat)
64 mg sodium
142 calories

KITCHEN TIP

Chicken Broth: Pour liquid through a sieve; discard the cooked vegetables. Freeze and use when chicken broth is called for in a recipe.

special occasions menu #4
Poached Chicken Breast

Poached chicken breasts become "gourmet" when served with **Cranberry Coulis** (page 215). Keep any extra sauce for another occasion.

2 cups	water	500 mL
1	bay leaf	1
2 tbsp	chopped onion	25 mL
2 tbsp	celery leaves	25 mL
Pinch	each: salt and pepper	pinch
4	boneless, skinless chicken breast halves (100 g each)	4

1 In skillet, bring water, bay leaf, onion, celery, salt and pepper to boil. Add chicken; cover and simmer for 15 minutes or until chicken is no longer pink inside. Remove from liquid; reserve liquid (see Tip).

2 Serve hot with our special **Cranberry Coulis**.

Makes 4 servings.

special occasions menu #4
Cranberry Coulis

Serve this sauce with **Poached Chicken Breast** (page 214). Chicken will become "gourmet" with this succulent sauce addition.

1/2 lb	fresh or frozen cranberries (see Tip)	250 g
1 cup	water	250 mL
4 tsp	lemon juice	20 mL
2 tsp	granulated sugar	10 mL
1	orange, peel and juice	1
2 tbsp	granular low-calorie sweetener with sucralose	25 mL

1 In medium saucepan, cook cranberries, water, lemon juice, sugar, orange peel and juice, over medium-low heat, for 8 minutes or until cranberries pop their skins. Press through a sieve or food mill. Stir in sweetener and refrigerate.

Makes 1 1/2 cups (375 mL) sauce—8 servings.

PREPARATION TIME:
10 minutes

COOKING TIME:
8 minutes

Each serving:
3 tbsp (45 mL) sauce

1/2 FRUITS & VEGETABLES CHOICE

6 g carbohydrate (1 g fibre)
0 g protein
0 g total fat
12 mg sodium
22 calories

KITCHEN TIP

A great time to make this sauce is when fresh cranberries are available in the fall. Prepare the sauce ahead and freeze to serve later.

PREPARATION TIME:
15 minutes

COOKING TIME:
30 minutes

Each serving:
1/2 cup (125 mL)

1 STARCH CHOICE
1/2 FATS & OILS CHOICE
1 EXTRA

22 g carbohydrate (**4 g fibre**)
2 g protein
2 g total fat (0 g saturated fat)
642 mg sodium
106 calories

KITCHEN TIP

Extra may be frozen in 1/2 cup (125 mL) serving sizes to reheat at a later time.

special occasions menu #4
Barley Pilaf

Ease the extra work of special occasions. Make this dish ahead of time and reheat in the oven or microwave just before serving.

2 tsp	soft margarine OR butter	10 mL
1 1/2 cups	sliced mushrooms	375 mL
1/3 cup	chopped onion	75 mL
1 cup	pearl barley	250 mL
2 1/2 cups	water	625 mL
2	chicken bouillon cubes OR sachets chicken bouillon powder	2
1/4 cup	chopped parsley	50 mL

1 In saucepan, melt margarine over medium-high heat. Add mushrooms and onion; sauté for 5 minutes or until softened. Add barley, water and chicken bouillon. Cover and cook for about 30 minutes or until barley is tender. Stir in parsley and serve. (See Tip.)

Makes 4 servings, 4 cups (1 L).

Strawberry Shortcake

Strawberry shortcake made with **Multimix** (page 36) is a lighter version of the traditional recipe that commonly uses a rich biscuit.

3	**Multimix Tea Biscuits** (page 185)	3
6 cups	sliced fresh strawberries	1.5 L
3/4 cup	whipped cream (6 tbsp/90 mL 35% cream)	175 mL
2 tbsp	liqueur, optional	25 mL

1 Split each biscuit in half. Place each half on individual serving plates.

2 Top each half with 1 cup (250 mL) strawberries. Whip cream with liqueur, if using. Spoon cream evenly over biscuits and strawberries.

Makes 6 servings.

PREPARATION TIME:
about 15 minutes if tea biscuits are ready

Each serving:
1/6 of recipe

**1/2 STARCH CHOICE
1 FRUITS & VEGETABLES CHOICE
1 1/2 FATS & OILS CHOICES
(2 FATS & OILS CHOICES with liqueur)**

19 g carbohydrate (4 g fibre)
2 g protein
8 g total fat (4 g saturated fat)
37 mg sodium
165 calories

PREPARATION TIME:
15 minutes

COOKING TIME:
40 minutes

Each serving:
2 pieces of chicken

1 STARCH CHOICE
4 PROTEIN CHOICES

16 g carbohydrate (0 g fibre)
31 g protein
10 g total fat (2 g saturated fat)
996 mg sodium
285 calories

special occasions menu #5
Crispy Baked Chicken

Seasoned dried bread crumbs provide a pleasantly crusty coating on tender chicken thighs or drumsticks.

12	small chicken thighs or drumsticks	12
1 cup	low-fat (1%) yogurt	250 mL
2 tbsp	Dijon mustard	25 mL
2 tsp	minced gingerroot	10 mL
1 cup	fine dried bread-crumbs	250 mL
2 tsp	garlic salt	10 mL
1/2 tsp	freshly ground pepper	2 mL
1/2 tsp	curry powder	2 mL
1/2 tsp	paprika	2 mL

1 Remove and discard skin and fat from chicken pieces.

2 In shallow dish, combine yogurt, mustard and gingerroot; set aside. In second dish, stir together bread crumbs and seasonings.

3 Dip chicken first into yogurt, then into bread crumbs. Place on baking pan sprayed with non-stick vegetable coating.

4 Bake in 350°F (180°C) oven for 40 minutes or until cooked and golden brown.

Makes 6 servings.

special occasions menu #5

Creamy Herb Dip

A blender or food processor makes short work of this recipe. Use the dip as both a salad dressing and as a dip.

1 cup	low-fat (1%) cottage cheese	250 mL
2/3 cup	low-fat (1%) plain yogurt	150 mL
1/3 cup	water	75 mL
2	green onions, chopped	2
1 tsp	Dijon mustard	5 mL
1/2 tsp	garlic powder	2 mL
1/2 tsp	dried basil leaves	2 mL
1/4 tsp	dried oregano	1 mL

1 In food processor or blender, process cottage cheese, yogurt and water until smooth. Pour into bowl and stir in onions, mustard, garlic powder, basil and oregano.

2 Cover and refrigerate for at least 30 minutes so flavours develop. Store in the refrigerator for up to one week. Stir before serving.

Makes 2 cups (500 mL).

PREPARATION TIME:
10 minutes

CHILL:
30 minutes or longer

Each serving:
1/3 cup (75 mL)

1/2 MILK 2% CHOICE

3 g carbohydrate (0 g fibre)
5 g protein
1 g total fat (1g saturated fat)
123 mg sodium
37 calories

PREPARATION TIME:
20 minutes

COOKING TIME:
5 minutes for vegetables

Each serving:
2/3 cup (150 mL) dressing

1 STARCH CHOICE
1 FATS & OILS CHOICE

16 g carbohydrate (1 g fibre)
3 g protein
5 g total fat (1 g saturated fat)
394 mg sodium
119 calories

KITCHEN TIPS

If you have bread-crumbs in the freezer, approximately 3 1/2 cups (875 mL) crumbs will replace 6 slices of bread.

To Stuff Poultry: Rinse and dry the cavity; stuff with prepared dressing. Close openings by trussing with a large needle and string or insert skewers and criss-cross the string. Cross legs over tail and tie with string so legs are close to the body. Turn wings back, tuck under the bird and secure with skewers or string.

To Roast Poultry: Place on rack in open roasting pan, breast side up, with a meat thermometer inserted in thigh. Roast in 325°F (160°C) oven until thermometer reaches 185°F (85°C) or juices run clear. If breast starts to brown too much, cover loosely with foil.

Poultry Dressing

Bread one to two days old makes the best dressing. Stuff poultry just before you roast it. This recipe stuffs a 6-lb (3 kg) chicken; double the recipe for a 12-lb (6 kg) turkey.

6	slices bread (crusts included)	6
2 tbsp	margarine or butter	25 mL
1 cup	chopped mushrooms	250 mL
1/2 cup	chopped celery	125 mL
1/3 cup	chopped onion	75 mL
1/4 cup	chopped parsley	50 mL
1 tsp	dried tarragon	5 mL
1/2 tsp	salt	2 mL
1/2 tsp	paprika	2 mL
Pinch	ground nutmeg and pepper	Pinch

1 Prepare bread-crumbs in food processor or by hand.

2 In a nonstick skillet, melt margarine on medium-high heat. Add mushrooms, celery, onion and parsley and cook for 5 minutes or until vegetables have softened. Cool, stir in seasonings and add to bread-crumbs. (See Tip)

Makes 6 servings, 4 cups (1 L)

special occasions menu #6

Braised Red Cabbage with Cranberries

The pleasing ruby-red colour and tart flavour of this unusual vegetable dish is a wonderful match with roast turkey.

1 tsp	olive oil	5 mL
1 tbsp	brown sugar	15 mL
3	large cloves garlic, crushed	3
1 cup	fresh or frozen cranberries, divided	250 mL
3 tbsp	red wine vinegar	45 mL
5 cups	shredded red cabbage (3/4 lb/375 g)	1.25 L
1/3 cup	dry red wine	75 mL
Pinch	cayenne pepper	Pinch
	Salt and pepper to taste	

1 In large saucepan, heat oil, brown sugar and garlic over medium heat for 2 minutes.

2 Add 1/2 cup (125 mL) cranberries and vinegar. Cover and cook for about 5 minutes or until cranberries pop their skins.

3 Add cabbage, wine and cayenne. Cover and cook on low heat for about 20 minutes or until cabbage is tender; stir occasionally.

4 Stir in remaining 1/2 cup (125 mL) cranberries. Remove from heat; cover and let stand for 5 minutes or until cranberries are warm. Season to taste with salt and pepper. Serve hot or cold.

Makes 8 servings, 4 cups (1 L).

PREPARATION TIME:
20 minutes

COOKING TIME:
about 30 minutes

Each serving:
1/2 cup (125 mL)

1/2 FRUITS & VEGETABLES CHOICE

6 g carbohydrate (1 g fibre)
1 g protein
1 g total fat (0 g saturated fat)
10 mg sodium
32 calories

KITCHEN TIP

A food processor makes short work of shredding the cabbage.

PREPARATION TIME:
10 minutes

CHILL:
30 minutes

Each serving:
3 tbsp (45 mL) raspberry sauce

1/2 FRUITS & VEGETABLES CHOICE

6 g carbohydrate (2 g fibre)
0 g protein
0 g total fat
12 mg sodium
23 calories

special occasions menu #6
Raspberry Sauce

Raspberry sauce over ice cream is the perfect lighter dessert following a holiday fowl dinner.

1	pkg (300 g) frozen unsweetened raspberries	1
1/2 cup	water, divided	125 mL
1 tbsp	cornstarch	15 mL
2 tbsp	granular low-calorie sweetener with sucralose	25 mL
1/2 tsp	almond OR orange extract	2 mL

1 In saucepan, cook raspberries and 1/4 cup (50 mL) water, covered, until raspberries are thawed and mixture comes to a boil.

2 Combine cornstarch, sweetener and 1/4 cup (50 mL) water; stir into raspberry mixture and cook until sauce thickens. Stir in almond extract. Cover and refrigerate for at least 30 minutes to cool.

Makes 1 1/2 cups (375 mL) sauce.

appendix 1

The ABCs of Nutrition and Diabetes

Amino acids are the building blocks that make up different proteins. There are at least 22 different amino acids in the proteins of the human body.

Antioxidants are substances in food that seem to protect the body against cancer and heart disease. Vitamins A, C and E act as antioxidants.

Beta carotene comes from dark green and yellow vegetables and fruits and is converted into vitamin A in the body. It is thought to act as an antioxidant.

Carbohydrates, found in grains, vegetables, fruits and milk provide energy for the body in the form of glucose. Carbohydrates are the part of a meal most responsible for raising blood glucose.

Cholesterol is a form of fat needed by the body to build cells and certain hormones. Most is manufactured in the liver. Some may come from animal food sources, but saturated fat is the main source of cholesterol. Too much cholesterol in the blood is linked to increased risk of heart disease. A total cholesterol/HDL ratio below 5.0 mmol/L is recommended.

Diabetes is a lifelong condition in which the body cannot properly store and use glucose fuel for energy. Insulin, a hormone produced by the pancreas, is needed in order for this to happen. (See *type 1* and *type 2* diabetes.)

Fatty acids are the building blocks that make up fats and oils. Most fat in foods is *triglyceride*, which consists of three fatty acids attached to a glycerol core. All fats are combinations of *saturated* and *unsaturated* fatty acids. Saturation refers to the amount of hydrogen a fatty acid can absorb.

Glucose is the simplest form of sugar, found in fruits and vegetables, and is the end result of starch digestion. Glucose circulates in the blood as the body's main source of energy.

Glucose monitors are small hand-held electronic devices that can estimate one's blood glucose level from a drop of blood placed on a sensor pad. The blood is obtained by pricking one's finger. Glucose monitoring at regular intervals makes improved diabetes control possible.

Glycemic index is a scale that compares the rise in blood glucose after different carbohydrate foods are eaten to the rise in blood glucose that occurs when the same person eats the same amount of carbohydrate as white bread or glucose. Slowly digested foods have a low glycemic index, while more rapidly digested foods have a higher glycemic index, closer to that of white bread.

Glycogen is a form of starchy carbohydrate stored in the liver and muscles. Liver and muscle glycogen both serve as reserves of glucose energy that can be released during periods of fasting or increased exercise.

Hypoglycemia occurs when blood glucose levels are lower than usual, usually below 3.5 millimoles per litre of blood. Normal blood glucose values are between 4 and 6 mmol/L. Usually only those using insulin or certain diabetes pills are at risk.

Monounsaturated fatty acids are found in olive, canola, peanut and avocado oils.

Omega-3 fatty acids are polyunsaturated fatty acids found in cold-water fatty fish. They not only help to lower blood cholesterol but also make blood platelets less "sticky" or likely to clot, thus reducing the risk of heart attack and stroke.

Polyunsaturated fatty acids are found in safflower, corn, sunflower and sesame oils.

Protein, the basic material of life, exists in many forms and is not intended to be an energy source. Muscles, organs, antibodies, some hormones and all enzymes are mostly protein. Proteins consist of chains of 22 assorted amino acids in different combinations. Some of these amino acids (the 10 *essential* ones) we get only from food, either directly from plant protein or indirectly from the protein of plant-eating animals. The rest can be manufactured in the body (so are *non-essential* in our diet).

Proteinuria is the abnormal loss of protein into the urine.

Saturated fatty acids are loaded with all the hydrogen they can carry. Fats containing a lot of saturated fatty acids are usually solid at room temperature. Most are animal fats, but both palm oil and coconut oils contain saturated fat. A diet high in saturated fat can result in high cholesterol levels and increased risk of heart disease or stroke.

Sodium is most familiar as part of sodium chloride, which we know as table salt. However, many commercial products have other kinds of sodium added to preserve them. Some people with high blood pressure or hypertension find it easier to control their blood pressure if they restrict their salt and sodium intake.

Sorbitol is sugar alcohol often used to sweeten dietetic candies and chocolate. It is more slowly digested than sugar. Too much at one time can cause cramping and diarrhea in some individuals.

Trans fatty acids are formed when hydrogen is added to the unsaturated vegetable oils used in the making of shortening and margarine. This *hydrogenation* makes them harder and more stable. These fats are used in many commercial baked goods and seem to be just as harmful as saturated fats in raising blood cholesterol.

Triglyceride is a kind of fat found in the blood, often measured at the same time as cholesterol. Too much (called hypertriglyceridemia) is also considered a risk factor for heart disease, especially in diabetes.

Type 1 diabetes is the less common form of diabetes usually but not always diagnosed before age 40. The pancreas either does not produce or produces very little insulin so that a person with type 1 diabetes is dependent on daily injections of insulin for life.

Type 2 diabetes is the type affecting 90% of those with diabetes. In this type, the pancreas can still make insulin, but the body doesn't use the insulin effectively. *Type 2* diabetes can sometimes be treated through diet and physical activity alone or in combination with medication and/or insulin injections.

Unsaturated fatty acids still have room for more hydrogen and are either monounsaturated or polyunsaturated. Fats containing these fatty acids are usually liquid at room temperature and come from plants and fish.

appendix 2

How to Use the Good Health Eating Guide (GHEG)

The Canadian Diabetes Association Food Choice System

This is a system that many people with diabetes use in planning meals and snacks. It is based on Canada's Food Guide to Healthy Eating with some changes to meet the needs of people with diabetes. Foods are divided into groups according to the amount of carbohydrate, protein and fat they contain. A serving of a food is described as a CHOICE, since it is your choice. By following a meal plan and choosing a variety of foods from each group, you're sure to get all the nutrients you need as well as having a consistent amount of carbohydrate and calories at each meal.

Starch Foods

These foods contain the carbohydrate you need for energy and also have a major impact on blood glucose. Many foods fit into this group. Most are low in fat and often high in fibre, but the amount you eat at any one meal matters. The *amount* of any starchy food described as 1 STARCH CHOICE contains 15 grams of carbohydrate (which ends up as about 3 tsp/15 mL of glucose sugar).

Breads and Rolls: You can choose any bread you like—they all fit into your meal plan—the trick is to know how much. One ounce (or 30 grams) of any bread item is equal to 1 STARCH CHOICE. Packaged breads, bagels, pita breads and so on clearly state the weight of one slice or one piece on the label. If your favourite bread or roll comes unpackaged, a small kitchen scale makes it easy to determine the weight.

Crackers and Breadsticks: There are many healthy high-fibre, low-fat, lower-salt varieties out there. Read labels. See how many crackers the label says are in a serving (usually a 30 gram portion), then compare the fat and fibre content (and sodium, if you're watching your salt intake). Because melba toasts, bread sticks and crackers contain less moisture than breads, 20 grams of crackers are equal to 1 STARCH CHOICE.

Breakfast Cereals: Like crackers, cereals are drier than bread, so 1 STARCH CHOICE usually equals a 20 gram serving. We've included a list of popular ready-to-eat breakfast cereals on page 233, showing the amount of each equal to 1 STARCH CHOICE.

Rice, Pasta and Legumes: A good rule of thumb to use is 1/2 cup (125 mL) cooked pasta or 1/3 cup (75 mL) cooked rice is equal to 1 STARCH CHOICE. With meat alternatives such as dried peas, beans or lentils, 1/2 cup (125 mL) cooked would count as 1 STARCH CHOICE plus 1 PROTEIN CHOICE. See your *Good Health Eating Guide* for more detail. Use a 1/2 cup (125 mL) OR 1/3 cup (75 mL) measure when serving starchy foods.

Starchy Vegetables: Potatoes and corn are classed as STARCH FOODS (even though we may think of them as vegetables).

Each of the following is 1 STARCH CHOICE:

1 slice bread (30 g)

1/2 English muffin (30 g)

1/2 cup (125 mL) cooked cereal

1/2 cup (125 mL) cooked couscous

1/2 cup (125 mL) cooked pasta

1 small OR 1/2 medium potato (95 g)

1/2 cup (125 mL) cooked quinoa

1/3 cup (75 mL) cooked rice

Fruits & Vegetables

We have used a wide variety of fruits and vegetables in our menus and recipes. Each choice from this group contains 10 grams carbohydrate. This could describe 1 small orange OR apple OR 1/2 small banana OR 1/4 papaya. This amount of fruit contains 10 grams of natural sugar and starch, and a variety of vitamins and minerals as well as fibre. Root vegetables and green peas are also in this group. Usually a 1/2 cup (125 mL) serving counts as 1 FRUITS & VEGETABLES CHOICE.

For your convenience, we have included a list of the fruits and vegetables we've used so that if you don't have the one named in the menu, you may replace with another and still get the same amount of carbohydrate.

Each of the following is 1 FRUITS & VEGETABLES CHOICE:

1 small OR 1/2 medium apple (75 g)

2 medium apricots (115 g)

1/2 small banana (without peel, 50 g)

1/2 cup (125 mL) blueberries (70 g)

2/3 cup (150 mL) cantaloupe (135 g)

10 cherries (with pits, 75 g)

1/2 small grapefruit (185 g)

1/2 cup (125 mL) grapes (75 g)

2/3 cup (150 mL) honeydew melon (115 g)

1 medium kiwi fruit (with skin, 76 g)

1 mandarin orange (with rind, 135 g)

1/3 cup (75 mL) mango (65 g)

1 small orange (with rind, 130 g)

1/4 medium papaya (without skin/seeds, 100 g)

1 large peach (with pit and skin, 100 g)

1/2 medium pear (with skin and core, 90 g)

1 slice raw pineapple (75 g)

1 slice canned pineapple in juice (with 2 tbsp/25 mL juice, 55 g)

1 medium OR 2 small plums (60 g)

2 stewed prunes (with 2 tbsp/25 mL liquid, 35 g)

1 cup (250 mL) raspberries (130 g)

1 cup (250 mL) strawberries (150 g)

1 wedge watermelon (with rind, 310 g)

1/2 cup (125 mL) carrots or beets

1/2 cup (125 mL) frozen peas

1/2 cup (125 mL) squash OR rutabaga

1 cup (250 mL) snow peas (135 g)

1 cup (250 mL) canned tomatoes

1 cup (250 mL) tomato juice

Milk

Milk and Yogurt: Low-fat or non-fat milk and yogurt are excellent sources of calcium and protein and good sources of riboflavin, phosphorus and vitamin B12. Our menus and recipes call for low-fat milk, which could be non-fat skim or 1%; we leave the choice up to you. The amount of milk sugar is the same; the only difference is in fat and calories. A small glass (1/2 cup/125 mL) non-fat skim has 40 calories; the same amount of 1% has 50 calories. Both contain 4 grams of protein and 6 grams of carbohydrate. And both would be called 1 MILK CHOICE. You may prefer to do as we do—drink skim and use it in cooking, and have 1% on hand to use on cereal and in tea or coffee. Your choice.

Lactose-Intolerance: Some people have difficulty digesting the lactose (milk sugar) in regular milk because they lack the necessary digestive enzyme. However, low-fat lactose-reduced milk is available in the dairy section of most supermarkets. It has the same nutrients and the same amount of carbohydrate and protein as regular milk, so a small glass still counts as 1 MILK CHOICE. Some prefer milk made from soya beans. If unsweetened, 1/2 cup (125 mL) soy milk is 1 MILK CHOICE. Read labels for fat and sugar content.

Cheese: Usually cheese is included in discussions of milk products. However, since cheese lacks the carbohydrate of milk, but contains protein and fat, it is found in PROTEIN FOODS.

Sugars

Sugars, and foods that contain added sugar, can be eaten in moderation by people with diabetes without upsetting diabetes control. The key is *how much* and *when*. Sugars should be spread throughout the day as part of slowly digested meals. The trick is to work it into a meal, not just add it on. For example, 1 SUGARS CHOICE is equal to 10 grams or 2 tsp (10 mL) sugar. 1 FRUITS & VEGETABLES CHOICE is also equal to 10 grams or 2 tsp (10 mL) sugar, so one could replace the other. Sugar could also replace one or more STARCH CHOICES. Our recipes carefully include any sugar as part of the total carbohydrate in a menu.

Protein Foods

This group contains meat and poultry, fish, eggs and cheese. One PROTEIN CHOICE is equal to 1 ounce or 30 grams of cooked meat. Each choice contains about 7 grams of protein and 3 grams of fat, although some choices may have more (or less) fat than this.

Meat is a good source of protein, but can contain too much saturated fat for heart health. Most of the fat in poultry is in or under the skin. Choose smaller portions, leaner cuts and trim well.

Fish and shellfish are also excellent sources of protein and are relatively low in calories and fat, especially saturated fat. Eating even one or two servings of fish a week is associated with a lower risk of heart disease. And the higher the fat content of the fish, the greater the "heart-healthy" benefits since fatty fish have the most omega-3 fatty acids. (see Appendix 1, page 224). Fish with a moderate- to high-fat content include bass, catfish, halibut, herring, mackerel, ocean perch, orange roughy, rainbow trout, salmon, sardines and smelt. Whitefish, cod, haddock and seafood are very low in total fat.

Eggs are an inexpensive source of quality protein as well as vitamins B12 and E. Eggs have been given an undeserved bad reputation as being high in fat and high in cholesterol. First of all, one egg yolk contains only 2 grams of saturated fat. Second, it is the saturated fat in food that is the main villain when it comes to causing heart disease, not the cholesterol in food. Four eggs a week is considered a reasonable limit.

Cheese: Like all dairy products, cheese is high in protein and calcium. It also tends to be high in saturated fat and sodium. However, some types of cheese are already low or moderate in fat (part-skim mozzarella, ricotta, low-fat cottage cheese). All cheese is marked with its fat content, so read labels and choose those with less fat (17% or less) as often as possible. Whenever we use cheese in a menu or recipe, we specify the weight in grams. Usually one ounce (25 grams) of cheese equals one PROTEIN CHOICE.

Meat Alternatives: Dried beans, peas and lentils are also excellent sources of protein. However, because of their carbohydrate content, they are listed as STARCH FOODS (see page 226).

Fats & Oils

One FATS & OILS CHOICE is equal to 5 grams or 1 teaspoon (5 mL) of fat (margarine or butter or oil) and has 45 calories. This group also contains foods high in hidden fat such as nuts and seeds. In a healthy diet, fats and oils should be used sparingly. Even though some are considered healthier than others, all contain a significant amount of fat and calories.

Margarine: A healthy margarine is a soft non-hydrogenated margarine, low in saturated and trans fat, and made from vegetable oils rich in monounsaturated fat, such as canola, olive, corn or sunflower. Light or diet margarine has been diluted with water to reduce calories so is not recommended for cooking or baking.

Butter: Butter contains the same amount of calories and fat as margarine, but most of its fat is saturated. However, if your diet is already low in fat, a little butter now and then won't hurt you.

Vegetable Oils: Olive, canola and safflower oils are all heart-healthy choices. The highest in monounsaturated oils are canola and olive (see page 6).

Extra Vegetables

Vegetables in this group contain only a small amount of carbohydrate but an abundance of vitamins, minerals and fibre. Use them often. A serving of 1/2 cup (125 mL) or less counts as 1 EXTRA VEGETABLE; a larger serving of 1 cup (250 mL) would equal 1 FRUITS & VEGETABLES CHOICE. See page 97 for more about vegetables.

Extras

Last but not least, there are many things that add flavour to our food. The term EXTRA means that one serving of any item in this group contains less than 2.5 grams carbohydrate and no more than 14 calories per serving. This group includes *Free Foods* that can be used without limit: beverages such as herbal teas, coffee, mineral water and diet pop; and seasonings and flavours such as herbs and spices, lemon and lime juice and non-nutritive sweeteners (see below). Also in this group are condiments that contain more carbohydrate and are "free" in *measured amounts only*. Examples are ketchup, no-sugar-added fruit spreads, barbecue sauce and so on. See the GHEG *Resource* for more information about how to use.

Non-Nutritive Sweeteners

There are different kinds and forms of sweeteners with different tastes and different uses. Some come in packets as tabletop sweeteners, others in tablets, others as liquids. All granular forms have a "filler" sugar to add bulk, so a maximum of three or four packets per day is suggested. Health Canada has approved all sweeteners listed below as safe for all Canadians. Generic name is listed first, followed by brand names.

- aspartame (Equal®, Nutrasweet®)
- cyclamate (Hermesetas®, Finesweet®, Sucaryl®, Sugar Twin®, Sweet'N Low® Sweet Magic®, Sweet-10®, Weight Watchers®)

- saccharin (Hermesetas®, Sweet 'n Low®)
- sucralose (Splenda®)

We have used a variety of sweeteners in our recipes and menus. However, we have used sucralose in all recipes that are cooked or baked with excellent results. Other sweeteners may lose sweetness or develop a bitter taste at high temperatures. In recipes where cooking is not required, use the sweetener of your choice.

The *Good Health Eating Guide Resource* contains more about sweeteners, reading labels, dining out, travel, and managing meals when you're feeling sick. GHEG pamphlets, posters and resource books are available from the dietitian at your hospital or diabetes education centre, at your local CDA Division office (see page 239) or at www.diabetes.ca.

appendix 3

Breakfast Cereals of Your Choice

Most prepared cold cereals are sweetened, but remember that it is *total carbohydrate* that counts. The *Good Health Eating Guide* defines the amount of cereal equal to one STARCH CHOICE as the amount containing 15 grams of carbohydrate (*not* including fibre). This is usually a 20 gram serving of cereal. To avoid guesswork, refer to the list below when you want to exchange one cereal for another in our menus. You will find most of these serving sizes to be smaller than the 30 gram serving size described on the cereal box.

1/2 cup (125 mL) All Bran™

1/3 cup (75 mL) All Bran Buds™

1/2 cup (125 mL) Balance™

2/3 cup (150 mL) bran flakes

1/2 cup (125 mL) 100% Bran™

1 cup (250 mL) Cheerios™

2/3 cup (150 mL) corn flakes

1/4 cup (50 mL) granola (low fat)

1/2 cup (125 mL) Just Right™

1 Muffet™ biscuit

1/2 cup (125 mL) raisin bran flakes

2/3 cup (150 mL) Rice Krispies™

1 shredded wheat biscuit

1/2 cup (125 mL) Shreddies™

1/2 cup (125 mL) Shredded Wheat Spoon-Size™

3/4 cup (175 mL) Special K™

appendix 4

Emergency Shelf Cooking

Too tired to cook? Not enough time to prepare recipes? Unexpected guests? These are the times for magic—the kind that an emergency shelf takes care of. Some suggestions for such a shelf (in your cupboard, refrigerator or freezer) follow.

Cupboard	Refrigerator	Freezer
canned soups	low-fat dips & spreads	ground beef or chicken
canned tuna, salmon, crab or shrimp, ham, baked beans in tomato sauce	**Make-Ahead Double Bran Muffin Batter** (page 45)	boneless chicken breasts or fish fillets, small lean steaks
light cheese spreads	low-fat milk, cream cheese, yogurt, sour cream	main courses
canned corn, tomatoes, fruit packed in juice	assorted low-fat cheeses	fruits frozen without sugar
pasta sauces	eggs	a variety of vegetables
assorted dry pastas & rice (preferably whole grain)	fesh fruits	single-serving lasagna
powdered skim milk	fresh vegetables	nuts
calorie-reduced gelatin & milk puddings with sweetener	salad greens & low-fat dressings	baked snacks
dried fruit	no-sugar-added fruit spreads	light ice cream
light peanut butter	mustard, salsa	
rolled oats		
dehydrated chicken/ beef bouillon		
several vinegars		

appendix 5

Stocking Your Refrigerator, Freezer and Cupboard

Do you ever get ready to cook, then go to the cupboard and find you are missing an ingredient? Here's a solution. The following is a list of extra ingredients to help make cooking more creative and certainly more fun. Keep on hand certain staples, like low-fat milk, all purpose flour, eggs, margarine or butter, salt, canned low-fat milk, sweeteners and sugar. Then look over our list of ingredients below, make your own list based on the menus you've chosen and then order or go shopping. In this way, you will be able to prepare a variety of the recipes in this book. We have indicated the best storage life for the following.

Refrigerator *Store for up to 1 week*	Freezer *Store for up to 3 months*	Cupboard *Store for up to 6 months*
lettuce green or red sweet peppers celery spinach green onions	fish (steaks or fillets) ground chicken, turkey or beef beef steaks veal cutlets pork or lamb chops	olive or canola oil brown/white rice light peanut butter breakfast cereals
Store for up to 2 weeks	*Store for up to 6 months*	*Store for up to 1 year*
grated parmesan cheese soft-style low-fat plain or herb cream cheese low-fat sour cream plain low-fat yogurt low-fat cheese carrots	boneless chicken breasts chicken pieces roasts vegetables cranberries dried fruits	long-grain rice vinegars light soy sauce canned soups canned broths assorted pastas

Refrigerator *Store for up to 2 weeks*	Freezer *Store for up to 6 months*	Cupboard *Store for up to 1 year*
cabbage eggs lemons	nuts	canned tomatoes canned vegetables diet soft drinks tea and coffee mineral water light hot chocolate light jelly powders sugar substitutes spices and herbs
Store for up to 1 month		
oranges apples lemons sun-dried tomatoes		
Store for up to 6 months		
no-sugar added fruit spreads light mayonnaise all mustards Worcestershire sauce horseradish dill pickles		

appendix 6

Nutrient Analysis of Recipes and Menus

Nutrient analysis of all recipes and menus chosen from *Choice Menus* was provided by Info Access (1988) Inc. using the Nutritional Accounting component of CBORD Menu Management System and the Canadian Nutrient File (1988) supplemented with data from the 1991 release. Nutrient analysis of recipes and menus chosen from *More Choice Menus* and *Choice Menus Presents* was carried out using the NUTRIWATCH Nutrient Analysis Program (1997), copyright to Elizabeth Warwick BHSc, based on the 1997 Canadian Nutrient File, and supplemented when necessary with documented data from reliable sources. Analysis was based on Imperial measures and weights (except for foods packaged and labelled in Metric amounts) and on the number of servings specified. Actual cooked weights were used where applicable.

Recipes were tested in both Imperial and Metric. Unless otherwise stated, recipes were tested and analyzed using canola or olive oils and soft margarine made from canola oil and 1% (2% in recipes originally from *Choice Menus*) milk and dairy products. Optional ingredients were not included in analysis. Microwave recipes were tested in a 750-watt, full-size microwave oven. If oven wattage is different, cooking times may have to be adjusted slightly.

Food Choice Values were assigned according to Canadian Diabetes Association guidelines (1994) with carbohydrate based on total carbohydrate minus dietary fibre. Total carbohydrate and dietary fibre are stated separately in recipe nutrient information. All recipe variations were analyzed and averaged only when ingredient food values were similar, otherwise separate Food Choice Values were assigned. All values were verified for the Canadian Diabetes Association by Katherine Younker, P.Dt. CDE in our first three books with additional recipes in this book verified by Sharyn Joliat, M.Sc. RD (Info Access).

Whenever appropriate, menus were analyzed using serving sizes specified in the *Good Health Eating Guide Resource* published by the Canadian Diabetes Association (1998). All canned fruit specified in menus and recipes refers to fruit canned in fruit juice.

Menus were planned to reflect current nutritional recommendations of the Canadian Diabetes Association: carbohydrate provides at least 50% of total energy; fat provides less than 30%, with 10% or less from saturated fat; protein about 20% of total calories. Monounsaturated oils were used whenever possible. All recipes state saturated fat in recipe nutrient information. Foods were selected for fibre content whenever possible and all recipes state total fibre content.

Each menu provides the following nutrients within a 10% deviation.

	Carbohydrate	Protein	Fat	Calories
Breakfast	46g	16 g	9 g	329
Lunch	59 g	24 g	12 g	440
Dinner	59 g	31 g	15 g	493
Total for Day	164 g	71 g	36 g	1264

Snacks:

75-calorie   10 to 15 g carbohydrate

150-calorie   15 to 20 g carbohydrate

300-calorie   35 to 40 g carbohydrate

appendix 7

Canadian Diabetes Association Area Offices

The Canadian Diabetes Association (CDA) is also an excellent source to obtain more information about diabetes and related issues.

Contact your area office, call the 1-800-BANTING line or visit the Association Web site (www.diabetes.ca) to find the branch closest to you.

PRAIRIES

Royal Bank Building
10117 Jasper Avenue NW, Suite 1010
Edmonton, AB T5J 1W8
Tel: (780) 423-1232
Fax: (780) 423-3322

PACIFIC

1385 West 8th Avenue, Suite 360
Vancouver, BC V6H 3V9
Tel: (604) 732-1331
Fax: (604) 732-8444

ATLANTIC

6080 Young Street, Suite 101
Halifax, NS B3K 5L2
Tel: (902) 453-4232
Fax: (902) 453-4440

ONTARIO REGIONS

1355 Bank Street, Suite 403
Ottawa, ON K1H 8K7
Tel: (613) 733-2634
Fax: (613) 733-5162

GREATER TORONTO/ CENTRAL SOUTH ONTARIO

235 Yorkland Avenue
Toronto, ON M2J 4Y8
Tel: (416) 363-0177 ext. 372
Fax: (416) 363-3393

NATIONAL OFFICE

522 University Avenue
Toronto, ON M5G 1Y7
Tel: 416-363-0177 OR
1-800-BANTING

Canadian National Institute for the Blind Information Source

The Canadian National Institute
for the Blind
1929 Bayview Avenue
Toronto, ON M4G 3E8
1-800-563-CNIB
www.cnib.ca

index